Chefs Can Save the World

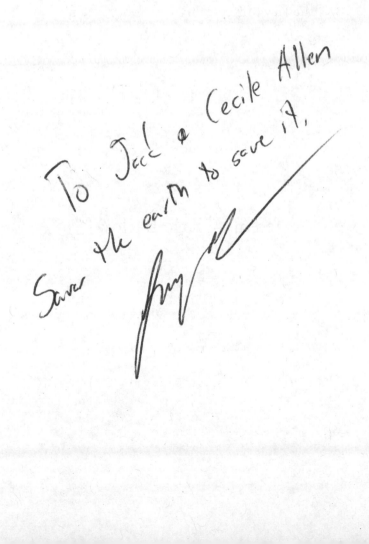

To Jack & Cecile Allen
Save the earth to save it,

Chefs Can Save the World

How to Green Restaurants and Why They Are
the Key to Renewing the Food System

Jeremy Chase Barlow

Printed in the United States of America

First Edition: October 2011

ISBN-13: 978-0-615-56962-8

ISBN-10: 0-615-56962-5

1. Health 2. Business

Dedication

This book is for my family,
immediate, extended, and professional.
You truly are the motivation
that drives me to achieve my goals.

Acknowledgements

I need to thank my wife and kids for providing me the time over the last three years to spend on this endeavor. There were times I thought it never would be finished. Thank you to my team: Adrien Matthews, William Gentry, Jason Lockman, and the rest of the crew at tayst who kept the ship running seamlessly; Cara Highsmith, my editor and English teacher, who kept me plugging away with nudging, offering constructive criticism and reinforcement along the way. She was an integral part in this project ever to come to fruition from the early stages over three years ago when the idea was in my head, to the step-by-step process along the way, and most of all to guiding the writing and the path. There is no possibility this book would have been finished without her; Mollie Henry who amazingly keeps my message out in the public and continually finds avenues of exposure; and my parents Dr. David and Beverly Barlow for offering help and guidance when needed along the way.

Contents

Introduction

What does it take to save the world? Is it possible to put the entirety—or even just the majority—of the human race on the path to a symbiotic relationship with Mother Earth? Can the innate "Darwinian" tendency for a human's fight for survival be tamed by one person, one group, or one profession? One would think the answer is overwhelmingly NO, but is it? The better question might be: *Does the world want to be saved?* Let's set this giant philosophical question aside and concentrate on the first question. *What does it take to save the world?*

Obviously, the first question asked of one hundred people will yield one hundred different answers. Therein lies the problem. The world has become so complicated with its global infrastructure of technology, trade, and politics that to attempt to fix it by attacking one issue is like plugging a hole in a dam with your finger. The leak will find another weak spot. Concurrently, the chance of looking at the overwhelming problems our world faces as a whole makes the will to face them weaker by the sheer magnitude of the situation.

Of course, none of this takes into account the first step of agreeing on the actual problems at hand, a seemingly impossible task. So let's pretend to agree on the path the world is on right now. Remove the religious differences, the bureaucratic road blocks, the worthless bickering by elected officials whose main goal, once elected, is to get reelected, and the myriad other obstacles preventing us from finding common ground. Throughout history we have used our intelligence to innovate, create, and destroy in order to build this world of global interaction. It seems we have reached an exponential growth cycle. The last one hundred years have seen the world shrink in an instant and its population increase by over 5 billion people.[1] The scientists focusing on the health of the planet are now starting to tell the same stories, whether it is regarding climate change, fossil fuels, water resources, air quality, land use, pollution, human health, etc.

The combined message is that we are quickly heading toward a time when our planet will be unable to provide us with the means to survive in the way we are accustomed. With the same speed that we shrank the world into a communications microcosm, we are quickly shrinking our natural resources and the raw materials that allow us to exist. If and when we run out of these limited resources we will not be able to stop and fix the problem. Once they are gone, they are gone. So we have to do the hardest possible thing for humans to do: think ahead, believe beyond our seeing, and plan for more than our immediate needs. We must try to fix the system that will eventually cause this "problem." And that brings us right back to where we started: What does it take to save the world?

There is an answer. It is the one act that binds all humans regardless of race, gender, geography, and religion. **We all need to eat.** By fixing the food system we can potentially alter the path of the world and truly look at a sustainable future.

Some historians say agricultural changes and advancements are at the root of our cultural development—it's the reason for the birth of cities, and the cause of wars. If these historians are correct, agriculture can again be the catalyst for the future of sustainability.

America has been the originator of many of these agricultural advancements and the understood leader of the developed world. But other countries have caught up with us, and in some cases, have flown right on by. Like the great civilizations of the past, it appears America has reached the apex of the bell curve and is on the way down. The issues the countries of the world face, by following our lead, are showing up in our country first: growing health concerns, dependence on fossil fuels, concerns about pollution, etc. Much of the rest of the world recognizes where this path is leading, knows there must be a change, and is looking toward alternate systems for the future. Other developing countries are following suit. That is why we are being surpassed. But it's not too late. We can get back on top of this world by leading the way in fixing these systems. Let's not, however, look at the whole world but focus on the (eco)systems within it—particularly the food system. It's the system with the most impact on this path of unsustainable living.

This fix is not going to happen if we depend on politicians, corporations, or the church. The answer can be found at the very place that made our country great: the hearth of America. In this day and age, the definition of hearth is different from what it used to be. Once, the hearth was the vital center of the home. But people don't stay at home anymore. They aren't going to slow down, put away their smart phones, and change this modern lifestyle that has taken hold. Yet they still have to eat. The new "hearth" is outside the home for the most part. The businesses currently in control of the food dollars are perfectly happy with the state of affairs, so they have no desire to change. They are making millions, if not billions, of dollars. We've all seen our government's inability to enact positive change surrounding any agricultural policies. Money makes the world go around, and nothing will change that. *The key is to change the money.*

The food system is the topic of many conversations right now. We will reiterate most of those discussions over the course of this book. Some in more detail than others, but it is important to show how many issues, economies, and people the food system involves. (The appendix to this book will include ample recommended resources to explore for more information.)

It is also important to understand how much power chefs wield within the food system. If we truly want to effect change in the food system, we need to change the money—how it's used, where it goes—and a good portion of the money moving through the food system is controlled by chefs.

Keep in mind I'm not talking about the fine-dining celebrity chefs you read about or even the restaurants like mine fortunate to be recognized for the attention they bring to the sustainable movement. Currently, most of these chefs are already involved in the sustainable food movement. I'm talking about the other 95% of chefs out there who are reaching a far greater portion of the community. Yes, I mean those who feed us on a daily basis, from chain restaurants and drive-thru windows, to cafeterias and hotel kitchens, to institutions and vending machines. They are the ones we need to reach.

I have a confession to make: My name is Jeremy Barlow, and I am an addict—a fast-food addict. I am not really sure how this addiction started. I grew up in a home with a mom who is a great cook. We had family dinners at the table most nights, and (possibly the most significant factor) for four months out of the year we lived on Nantucket—an island with no chain restaurants or fast-food places. There isn't even a stoplight. For me, Stuart MacKenzie from the movie *So I Married an Axe Murderer* said it best:

"Oh, I hated the Colonel with his wee beady eyes, and that smug look on his face . . .

Oh, you're gonna buy my chicken! Ohhhhh!"

"How can you hate the Colonel?" says Charlie.

"Because he puts some kind of chemical in the chicken that makes you crave it fortnightly, smartass!"

Ironically, this comedic quote holds a lot of tragic truth. I am not sure how it happened; but, for more than a third of my life I ate fast food for probably 60–70% of my meals. Oddly, a good portion of that time I was training to be a chef. I believe I ate it for the same reasons most Americans turn to this option: time and money. We live in a fast-paced society where the emphasis is on working, and working a lot. Restaurant folk are no different. In fact, the restaurant industry probably demands more hours for less pay than most other fields out there. We endure this because we love food.

I am happy to say I have been almost completely fast–food-free since I started writing this book. I used to dip tobacco as well, a nasty habit. It is a toss-up on which habit was harder to kick, but I am going with fast food. It's pretty amazing to me that fast food could be harder to quit than tobacco. My palate prefers salty and crunchy—not at all uncommon—and these are two key components of fast food . . . still, you'd think I'd struggle more with a nicotine addiction than my dependency on this greasy junk food. Although that does bring up some questions about the eerily similar nature of the corporate, industrialized food system and the tobacco industry, particularly the secrecy with which the industry operates. An excellent article examining these connections appeared in the *Milbank Quarterly* in the spring of 2009. It reported, "The food industry differs from the tobacco industry in several important ways, but uses some of the same strategies to respond to concerns about the health consequences of their products."[2] Even chefs who guard special ingredients when sharing a recipe will at least give you an idea of what's in a dish, but getting full disclosure from these companies is nearly impossible.

So, will I ever have fast food again? Probably. It's also likely I'll take my kids through a drive-thru on a road trip one day; but, for the most part, I no longer crave it. Even when I have the occasional urge I find myself being turned off as I come close to getting it. It is almost like the small part of my brain that causes my craving is overridden by my body's reluctance to endure the repercussions of eating it.

There are a couple reasons I think so many people eat fast food, but the main one is that it tastes good. Do we have a religious experience with each bite we take? No. But, the fact is, it is consistently pleasing and, possibly most compelling, it's cheap. With the exception of produce (which is another discussion) that's basically the key to the entire industrialized food system. The fast-food system and the industrial food system are relatively interchangeable, and it's not difficult to see how the demands of the fast-food industry pushed the rapid development (possibly the destruction) of the industrial food system. Any product, whether it's processed, ground, or baked, is manufactured to look, feel, and taste the same everywhere it is sold. In addition to making those flavor profiles easy to replicate, they are designed and manufactured to be cheap. The last significant reason fast food is king is its convenience. We work too hard, too long, and do way too much, thus, eating choices are more often than not based on speed and ease.

Regardless of the effects on our environment from supplying a nation with a multitude of processed food options, and regardless of how many people know these options are bad for them, fast food and/or industrialized food will continue to be in demand. Throughout this book we will explore some of the negative aspects of the industrial food system and the resulting connections between those effects and a number of the issues we face as a society. However, you might be surprised to see that I do not propose total elimination of fast food. Not only is that an unrealistic goal, it is counter-productive to try to remove those options completely. Instead, we should be educating people to make healthy, safe, and responsible choices. Our emphasis should be on intensive education efforts toward the individuals purchasing the majority of the food in this country, encouraging them to request local, eco-friendly options. In addition, we need to begin training the next generation about the right choices through the food served in our schools. We have to promote healthy living from an early age instead of serving flavored milk, nutritionally reinforced donuts, Pop-Tarts, and processed shapes with chicken in them. I hope this book will show those in the fast-food industry that they *can* operate in an environmentally friendly manner, serving healthy, real food, and that they will reap benefits from this practice. There is nothing wrong with some eco-chic drive-thrus. The corporate food world has already shown us they are more than willing to provide us with what we want: fast, convenient, cheap, and tasty. It boils down to basic supply-and-demand economics. If we increase the demand for quality products, we can force an increase in the supply. Increased supply will make the healthier products more financially accessible, and corporate food companies will rise to meet the demand because they want a piece of that financial pie.

I am a cook, a comment I repeat often in this book, and do so for a specific reason: to clarify my position. I don't have advanced degrees in environmental studies or agriculture. I don't really have much of a science background at all. What I do have is a passion for food. Everything I believe about food that I have developed over the last few years and discuss in the following pages were shaped by some of the recent voices exposing the truth about the state of our industrial food system. People such as Michael Pollan, Eric Schlosser, Brian Halweil, Gary Hirschberg, and Joel Salatin were integral in changing my views not only on how I do my job, but how I live my life. These authors, along with Wendell Berry, Marion Nestle, Joan Gussow, and a few others were the trailblazers in reporting how food gets to the table and the results of that process. Everything they revealed and explained made sense to me. Most importantly, I could see it with my own eyes every time I looked in the mirror. Controlling my weight since graduating from college has been a constant battle, and it's completely related to my diet, how much I work, and how little I exercise, and maybe a few too many beers (don't let my wife know I'm admitting that one).

In this book my goal has been to take the information these authors have made available and apply it to the world of restaurants without just regurgitating the same data, although that is inevitable for some discussions. In fact, I will try to focus mainly on the basics of the issues we face in our food system and how they relate to restaurants. I want to spark in you the desire to personally delve into the issues and to really understand what is at stake by showing how it relates to the restaurant business; but, as you'll find, it also relates to your home, your community, and the environment. We will discuss frequently debated issues, such as school food, because they are a part of the equation. The one universal connection between all the research on sustainability and the issues raised in these discussions is the current food system. Since we, as a culture, spend 50% of our food budget outside the home presenting this in the context of a restaurant is the most effective medium. We are talking about $600 billion per year being controlled by food purchasers who more than likely are or were a cook or chef at some point. Additionally, we are experiencing the phenomenon of the celebrity chef, and by combining the public's interest in restaurants with this push for local, sustainable food, I've found a venue for passing along the valuable lessons I've learned.

Listening to these voices, while simultaneously building a purchasing infrastructure for becoming 100% local, was my impetus for delving further. Eventually, what I discovered inspired me to take my restaurant from "farm-to-table" to "green." Farm-to-table is a great start, but it is only a part of the footprint of the restaurant. I truly believe that if you participate in farm-to-table for the right reasons you will start to look at the whole restaurant from a green point of view. This was no easy task, and I decided to go further by becoming certified through the Green Restaurant Association (GRA)—a non-profit group started in 1990 with years of experience assisting restaurants in lessening their carbon footprint. For years they were the only group to do this. Now there are a few non-profits in the country certifying restaurants; however, there are also many for-profit groups offering certification assistance in order to peddle their wares. For me, the jury is still out on whether that is detrimental to the cause. Ultimately, I think any green steps you take will have a positive impact on your community and the environment, and, therefore, are a good thing. As in all areas of this green business wave, people are taking advantage of the public's general concern to leave the world a better place. Whether you are currently a restaurateur, an up-and-coming cook, or serious foodie, when this book, hopefully, inspires you to green your own restaurant or kitchen or influence others to do so, be careful to do the due diligence in investigating the organization you choose to assist you.

Most of the discussions out there right now regarding our food system deal with sourcing food—knowing where your food comes from and how it's grown—and ensuring a sustainable food system. But what is a sustainable food system? Is there a definitive, widely accepted answer available right now? No. In all the sustainable food circles this debate continues, much like the debate on climate change. You can look at the science that tells you what is good and what is bad from an environmental, health, and economic perspective, but you must also use common sense. Pay attention to your surroundings as you ingest this information. My definition of sustainability is this: a food system that provides everyone with a healthy, nutritious, and affordable diet without harming the environment in any way, while continuing to be fruitful indefinitely.

Is that possible or even realistic? Or should we simplify the answer to be a system that can just continue to grow food indefinitely. This is what we will work to determine. At some point we could find that answer in science—fertilizers and chemicals. Maybe it's a system in which all food is bought locally. But these answers only bring up more questions. For example: Couldn't food grown farther away with centralized shipping be easier on the environment than the impact of consumers and farmers driving to the farmers' markets? Let's break it down even more. Define just sustainability: policies and strategies that meet society's present needs without compromising the ability of future generations

17

to meet their own needs.[3] However, that is a vague definition, and as you get into the complexities of how that definition is applied it becomes much hazier. There is no easy answer. Since restaurants control a major portion of the dollars spent on food, would all restaurants then be required to green their operations in order to have a sustainable food system? I think so. As you enter the sustainability discussion from a restaurant's perspective you will discover how wasteful the commercial food industry is. This is really where it is crucial to pay attention to your surroundings. You will learn that 15% of food served comes back to the kitchen and that each meal produces one-and-a-half pounds of waste. An individual restaurant will produce 50,000 to 100,000 pounds of waste a year; a fast-food restaurant produces 200 pounds of waste for every $1,000 sold.[4] The most astonishing fact: 95% of this waste is recyclable. The average restaurant uses 300,000 gallons of water per year. The industry is responsible for one-third of the energy usage in the retail sector. These numbers are impossible to imagine and should be shocking enough to make everyone want to change.

I didn't just wake up one day and see the light. Okay, maybe I did, but what made it click for me as a way of life was the cumulative effect of revelations that came daily from doing my job as a chef. It started as a quest for the best ingredients in order to improve my cooking; but, what awakened in me was recognition of the importance for change in my entire operation. Through the experiences I share I hope not only to encourage you to . . . I hate to say follow in my footsteps because I don't see myself as a trailblazer, so, maybe . . . investigate the importance of greening your restaurant and act on it, or to demand this from the restaurants you patronize. I also hope to provide some useful resources to help inform your perspective. There are consultants out there who can be effective in helping you accomplish these goals; but, to have the perspective of someone who has been through it provides insight I feel is important to share.

Really, what does all of this sustainability mean for restaurants? Is "farm-to-table" a marketing tool? Is "greening" a gimmick? What does the obesity epidemic have to do with how I run my business, what my candles are made from, and what we feed our kids? These are questions I will try to answer. One other reason I have decided to share my stories is that at my restaurant we have been successful in significantly decreasing our carbon footprint without using a lot of money. We have had to be creative in the steps we have taken—and are continuing to take. Affordability is a serious fear, and a deterrent, for a lot of people, when the truth is, it can be done without a great deal of expense. What you will find out by the end of this book is that by wisely using the funds you do have available, a few selectively spent dollars will save you more money in the long run. Also, it could make you money. Almost 80% of diners say they prefer patronizing a certified green restaurant.[5]

I think the most important and rewarding result from the recent path toward a more sustainable restaurant is the increased involvement in my community. One of the greatest by-products of focusing your sourcing efforts locally is the benefit your community will receive. There is a very real connection between sustainable practices and the life of your community. There is a not-so-insignificant secondary consideration as well: the global ramifications. When you look beyond just the acquisition of food to the results of how it's grown, you see the connections. You realize that by making a sustainable local community you can affect the global one as well. You see that things happening on the other side of the world have an effect on your neighborhood and vice versa. This is equally evident in the industrial food system as we rely more and more on food grown far away. You realize that the ecosystem as a whole is very fragile and completely connected to the food system. You could say that the hearth is the heart of the Earth.

As a chef/owner I get pulled in a lot of directions, so I learn as I go. I don't typically have time to sit and research for hours; so, as I put my experiences into words, I needed to gather even more evidence about our situation. Mark my words, we are definitely in a dire situation. Everyone has felt it or seen it over the last few years. You can't turn on the news or read the paper without seeing some social issues troubling our communities—the economy, health care, climate change, and national security, to name a few. For the sake of time we will focus solely on the connections with restaurants, but the path our society is on has few happy endings and many bad ones. What became clear as each piece of the puzzle fell into place is that almost all of our problems are tied to the food system— and the key to unraveling the issues and achieving the solution is to fix the system, not the problems it causes.

There are two approaches to fixing our food system: bottom-up and top-down. Bottom-up is happening right now. Farmers' markets are increasing. People are requesting local and sustainable products in every facet of life—from their restaurants to their schools. Small businesses are taking the green path, and restaurateurs are starting to realize that they can play a significant role in making a difference. Top-down is happening, albeit at a slower rate, such as open discussions of policy changes, the U.S. Department of Agriculture (USDA)'s new school nutrition act, the potential changes to the farm bill, and the White House garden, among others. I think the best answer lies somewhere in the middle. Again, the fact is that money rules the world, and as long as the multinational corporations are controlling the system, things will remain status quo. They will spend millions to keep the policies stagnant because they stand to make tens of millions, if not billions, of dollars. The other reality is that, even though this movement is receiving lots of attention, the majority of people are not going to become involved. Accessing sustainable products, for those who care to, is very difficult for most of the population for myriad reasons. I think the best solution is found in the cooks and the chefs of our communities. With the number of dollars they control, they have the ability to insist these corporations do more than add organic options. They have enough buying power to change the way food is grown in order to meet their demands. One fact is certain, corporations will change to meet demand. As evidenced by the mechanization of the industrial food system that was brought about largely by corporations and the fast-food industry, chefs can reverse the trend and force corporations to go back (and push forward) to a successful system that includes sustainable food and methods. A sustainable food system will be enough to alter the path of all the systems. **Chefs *can* save the world.**

So what is the purpose of this book? I hope to show anyone involved in the restaurant community, and even those who are just interested in it, the importance of paying attention to where their food comes from and that it is possible to change. I want to show the connections between the food systems and almost every aspect of our culture and the impact that even one restaurant can have. I hope to add some clarification to the definition of sustainability from a restaurant point of view. I want to provide hands-on experience for the how and why of greening restaurants and the importance of doing so. Probably most importantly, I want to show how chefs truly have an ability to make a huge difference, not just in the food system as we know it, but in the ability to ensure a sustainable food system for the generations to follow—to ensure that our grandchildren can eat real food.

First tāyst

Chapter One
Passion

As I sit in front of a computer to put into writing the most recent years of my life, I find it incredibly ironic that one of the reasons I chose my profession was because it kept me from sitting at a desk researching, reading, and writing. I happen to love reading; but, my wandering mind, and probably some form of Attention Deficit Disorder (ADD), make it a challenging task. This, combined with a little bit of an addictive personality is, I think, why I was drawn to cooking, or at least in the beginning, why cooking suited me. The fast-paced, action-filled work environment, the shit-talking, hard-partying cooks, and basic disregard for self were right up my alley. By disregard for self I mean the all-out sacrifice to get through the night and make sure the customer is happy. Burns, cuts, wipeouts, and the all-too-common hangovers never slow you down. No real cook calls in sick, you get sent home. Never let the team down. The kitchen draws a certain type of personality, and, for whatever reason, I am that type.

I often wonder what the underlying link is between cooks. You can take a cook out of ten different kitchens, put all of them in one place, and after a few days they will connect like they have been working together for years. I guess it's the basic question of nature versus nurture. Just like most arguments regarding nature versus nurture, or the ones I can remember from my psych classes, this one has no definitive answer. It takes both to be a good cook. Fifty percent is nurture. You learn through training, school, books, TV, and the Internet, all the while getting better through practice. Fifty percent is nature. I think that this half is made up of two primary components. First, you have to have a solid work ethic. This goes beyond the ability to show up on time and work your fifteen-hour day. Someone with a good work ethic is always looking for that little bit extra they can give. You have respect for the entire work environment, not just your little corner of the restaurant. If you're walking inside from the parking lot and see trash, you pick it up. If you see a mess in the bathroom, you don't just ignore it. A strong work ethic is picking up your line mate's *mise en place* (daily preparations) when they need help. You pay attention to the little details, like making sure a small dice is a small dice.

The other aspect of nature, and the essential foundation for any good cook, whether amateur or professional, is passion. You can't teach passion. You can't learn passion. Passion is something that exists within you and is brought out by certain events or actions. In some way or another passion is in everybody, just like the need to eat, and it is discovered and it evolves as we go through life. As a child the passion might be for swimming in the waves, sports, reading, dancing, etc. As we get older, those passions go beyond one's self-interests to include people, careers, quality of life. Do you remember sitting out under the stars with *the one*, the sensation of their touch on your arm? You didn't feel it just around your arm, but breathed it in with the night air and it overcame your whole body. As we grow up we tend to follow the path made up of things we love. We marry those who inspire the most passion in us; we concentrate on the activities that provide the most enjoyment; and we live in places that give us comfort. Hopefully, if we're smart, we even choose a career that is emotionally and intellectually fulfilling, rather than just choosing a place to work and get a paycheck. That is not to say we don't stray or find ourselves in situations in which we thought we really loved something that, in reality, wasn't meant to be. There are also people who choose to follow money, or a path that was chosen for them and that seems impossible to change.

FINDING YOUR PASSION

Cooks are individuals who follow their passion. No one cooks for money or fame; and, if that is your goal, get out now because there is no money in it and fame only lasts for fifteen minutes—if you are lucky enough to get it. This reminds me of an article I read a long time ago covering an interview with an up-and-coming celebrity, a top-notch chef, who was asked about his fame. He made the comment that for every one of him there were six or seven other chefs as good as or better than he who will go unnoticed.

The aspect of passion in this profession—although I believe there is an important place for it in every profession—is vital because you cannot put out good food if you don't love what you are doing. You don't stay in a field requiring countless fifteen-hour days on your feet in cramped, windowless spaces with people screaming at you constantly unless you love it. You don't miss every wedding, family event, or holiday unless you love it. You don't give up every weekend unless you love it. You don't come home from work to read food books while watching food shows unless you love it. If you choose to be a cook—a good one at that—you eat (pun intended), sleep, and live food. The way you cook becomes an extension of you, and, in turn, your passion. The two are linked, and it's easy to tell the difference between a cook who cares and one who is going through the motions.

We cook from within; and, therefore, our food reflects our moods and our feelings. Personal bad days are rough to endure in the kitchen. Most good cooks can overcome them, but it takes much more work to get that special something extra out of a cook in a bad mood. I've been known to take cooks off the line to try to break them out of their mood; otherwise their food will not be as good. But for good cooks, even in bad moods, the food is revered above all else. As I put these sentiments on paper it sounds kind of fanciful, but it's true. If you ever get a chance to stand in a kitchen when a farmer walks in with their spoils, or when fish that was in the water the day before is delivered (we are landlocked in Nashville, Tenn.), it's an amazing sight. All work stops—albeit for only a second, but it does stop—because the cooks come over to check out the product. They look, smell, touch, and even taste when possible, to take in what has been delivered. This excitement for the rewards of the earth never ends and never gets old. This is the essence of the passion that cooks have. It's really pretty amazing. A strawberry, a radish, some arugula—they're basically sun, water, and soil, but so different and taste so amazing, unless, of course, they have been shipped a thousand miles first. Then they don't taste like anything.

This belief about the passion for food really solidified for me when I took my staff and my family to a farm operated by one of my friends. I would describe him more and tell you about the farm; but, he is the "farmer who must not be named," as he is the most famous guy in our city who doesn't want to be famous. Finding someone in Nashville who doesn't want to be famous is pretty amazing. In fact, I think one of the local food critics has a reward out for any information on his whereabouts.

That Sunday afternoon we walked around the farm pulling vegetables out of the ground, talking about how they were grown, the rotation of the crops, the reintroduction of nutrients, while wiping off the dirt and tasting them. It was an enlightening experience. I had been using more and more local food over the previous couple of years, but even that didn't compare to the flavors these veggies had right out of the ground. It was as if I was sitting at one of the best restaurants in the world, eating the best meal of my life cooked by Escoffier himself. As one of my good regulars said one night: "This is drop-your-fork good." After fifteen years of cooking, I finally knew exactly how a carrot was supposed to taste. I recognized the natural sweetness underneath the bite of the turnip. The list of all the great veggies we tasted that day goes on and on. That was the day I became solely dedicated to cooking with as much local product as I could. To work toward an infrastructure of supply that could eliminate the need for food from "far, far away." Of course, there are exceptions: products such as fish, oils, and certain spices indigenous to places outside our area that are required for certain types of cuisine. However, my passion for food, cooking, and pleasing guests could not allow me to rob them of the wonderful flavors you get from a freshly picked vegetable. It seems like a pretty basic concept, but you'd be surprised by how hard it is to stick to that principle. That is how far we have come in the last fifty years. More than 2,000 years of eating from our backyard have devolved into a need for an underground movement of like-minded people to bring the importance of local food back to the forefront. The power of this movement is growing at a viral rate; but, it is still a movement, and in order to fully engage in a sustainable food system, it needs to become second nature. Even though, in actuality, it is first nature.

PURSUING YOUR PASSION

I say I started to use local food as much as I could as often as I could because it's not that I couldn't run a restaurant with 100% local food. I could. Well, in the beginning I couldn't, but that ability was definitely in the foreseeable future. There was another underlying issue in this newfound goal of 100% local that made me hesitate in the beginning. A restaurant is still a business; and, to an extent, I can't deny the customers what they want—it is a service industry after all. If I wanted to stay in business, I had to tread a line between (for lack of a better term) steak and potatoes and more adventurous offerings. To those in foodie cities—where, if the food and service are good, the more creative the better—this may seem like a pretty crazy concept. The reality is that only a small segment of the population is ready for pig heads and hearts—nose-to-tail cookery. In Nashville, which I feel is a great example of the typical mid-sized American city, we still are not quite ready for that on a large scale. If we are really looking for the successful integration of a sustainable food system, we have to appeal to everyone. Here is a perfect example: Five years ago I couldn't give away the pork belly dish on my menu. Now, we can't go through enough pig to keep it in stock. We are also selling dishes like heart, head cheese, and lamb fries like they're going out of style. We have reached the point where we can run a menu with no greens and guests don't look up and say, "What, you don't have any salads?" People are beginning to comprehend—or remember—that certain food isn't available all year long. Our demographic—a small percentage of the city—understands our philosophy and what we serve.

Also, there are some foods I couldn't live without, seafood being one of them, and olive oil is another—items that aren't local to Nashville. So this became my motto: *Do As Much As You Can, As Often As You Can.* It's not that initiatives like "Eat Local" and the 100-mile diet can't be done all the way. They have been, and are continuing to be done, with a full commitment; but the reality of making it happen becomes more realistic on a grander scale when you don't set hard and fast rules. There is nothing wrong with eating local in any percentage. In fact, when the approach is made so absolute, I feel it turns people off of what you're trying to accomplish. You can't force people, but you can inspire them to change a little at a time.

My passion fueled this initial evolution, but didn't stop when I first made the effort to buy locally. It didn't stop when I had found the two or three farms selling locally at that time. In fact, I began to wonder if *Do As Much As You Can, As Often As You Can* was a rationalization. I started to view it as a cop-out. *Do as much as you* can evolved into *do everything you can.* My passion grew and became infectious. As I learned more about sustainability, I began to set parameters for my definition of sustainability, and as I built a functional infrastructure of supply, we inherently became more local. We are always striving to do more.

Besides, when you really get into the benefits of local food, as I will discuss later, there is one primary aspect that stands out above all others for why it is the better choice, for why passionate cooks will choose it almost every time: It just tastes better!

When you break it down, passionate cooks all over the world care about one thing: How does it taste?

Chapter Two
Evolution

I think I should give a little history so you can have some insight on how I got to this point of my cooking life, which will hopefully show how easy and natural that change can be.

I had never really taken the time to evaluate my cooking style before starting this project. I now feel defining my style serves an important purpose. In hindsight, I see I've followed a very specific path—the evolution of my food and how I became determined to embrace sustainable farming and a sustainable business—on the journey to being green.

In fact, when I first decided to take the restaurant green and proceeded to make it public, I stated in a couple of interviews that I wasn't an activist. I just thought I could be an example. I hoped to show people that green is possible and hoped they would follow; but, I had no intention of walking around with my hippie-stick preaching the green gospel. The reality is I only knew a little about the green movement at that time. Even now, I feel as though I have only scratched the surface of the information regarding the impact on the environment created by the restaurant industry, the current food system, and our culture. Somehow though, I knew it was the right move. I was convinced it was the only way to operate a restaurant. The passion I feel for the things I value is rivaled only by my passion for food, therefore, I found myself dragged somewhat reluctantly into the role of activist. The more I learn about the condition of our world and the food we produce, the more I find myself pushing for changes in our legislative policies, in our school systems, and in general public awareness. I have come to terms with this new identity, and I try to do it without getting on my soapbox, but there are still hot-button issues (any issue related to the food system), that get me going. The one thing that helped me to accept this newfound activism was one of my first experiences at culinary school. During a welcome speech by Ferdinand Metz (after an excellent display of how little we all knew), he said something that has really stuck with me. To sum it up, he said chefs determine the direction of the food trends in the country through their exposure in the media, the food they serve in their restaurants, and the recipes they put into magazines and books. This was before the phenomenon of the celebrity chef really crept into homes across America, so that was not an element he addressed in his speech. However, now more than ever, with the chef as a celebrity, we have the power to change trends in our industry. Fortunately, I don't see the sustainable food movement or the future of green restaurants being held to the ebb and flow of a trend.

TREND FOLLOWER OR TREND SETTER?

In every trend there are aspects that are more than just a fad and tend to outlive the trend itself. This is a trait specific to industries involving artisans: woodworkers, designers, cooks, etc. They are also the industries in which trends reflect the current desires of the masses. Cooks are craftsmen. They create and replicate dishes over and over. Really good cooks are able to make a dish exactly the same every single time it is made. These dishes, especially in the beginning, are influenced by the people who are eating them. It starts in the kitchen with the first taste and subsequent comments. Then the staff samples and offers their opinions, next it might go to a few regulars, and finally to the menu. The remarks sink in, and consciously or subconsciously, they affect the final form the dish takes. Obviously, there are exceptions—those who have reached the point of mastering their craft and those who refuse to listen. In most cases, when you create dishes and menus and offer them up to the public, you get feedback. This feedback will inevitably affect your views or thoughts on the next creation. I guess if you locked yourself away in the kitchen and spoke to no one, you could escape being influenced by external points of view; but as I said before, this is a service industry, and we work to provide others with a great experience. It doesn't matter whether it's with the family at a chain restaurant throwing peanut shells on the floor or at a three-star Michelin restaurant, the goal is to please your customers.

The major food trends I've dabbled in throughout my career have been Pacific Rim, Fusion, Comfort (not really a trend but more of a fallback in between trends), Southwestern, and the latest, Molecular Gastronomy. I really like this one because it fits my playful side, although I have never really been able to completely explore it due to the expense involved in all the high-tech gadgets necessary to be really successful with it. Nor have I had a kitchen staff large enough to execute it properly. However, I have definitely taken opportunities to sneak in some of these space-food techniques. This is the remarkable thing about a trend. Individuals take aspects of each trend, learn through experience, and personal styles are developed. Some people cook all Fusion, some all Southwestern, some vary their style within a genre; but in my experience, most young cooks working their way up the ladder take a piece of each style and add it to their arsenal. As the time comes for them to start developing their own food styles they draw on these experiences and turn them into something all their own. At least that is what happened with me.

I call my cooking style "Playful American." It's not really a designation I've heard before, but it really fits what we try to do. As you know by now, we use as many local sources for food as we can—right now, anywhere from 80% to 95%—and we serve it with a twist on a classic dish or a play on words in order to make it fun. We place no boundaries on what we do when it comes to combinations or flavor profiles. As long as it tastes good and it puts a smile on our faces, we will put it out. My belief is people want to have fun when they go out. I also believe that can start as early as the descriptions on the menu. It's basic psychology (with a touch of logic): If you are having fun and guests see you having fun, guests will have fun. The crucial component is being able to deliver on what you promise; otherwise you're only amusing yourself. When the guests leave, they will take away a good vibe and a positive experience, which will make them more likely to return.

LEARNING THE ROPES

I will trace for you the path of how I came to cook like this, how my cooking came to reflect my personality. How did I get to the point in which I chose to make the restaurant business harder?

I went to cooking school in Hyde Park, N.Y. But the experiences that most molded me as a person and definitely shaped my cooking style happened on Nantucket where I grew up. I started washing dishes when I was seventeen and moved up to cooking pretty quickly. That restaurant was, and remains to this day, one of the coolest places I've ever worked. The White Dog Café—part café, part college bar, and part movie theater—offered food that was pretty straightforward. During my second summer I was able to try making a few of their dishes, and even put some together on my own. Lime chicken quesadillas, *ridiculously* hot wings—dishes a twenty-year-old college kid would want to eat. The dishes seem simple now, but since I was just starting out, it took me all day to make them, not to mention another day to clean up. Why is it that learning how to work cleanly is just as hard as learning how to cook? Anyway, it wasn't the food there that hooked me. It was the lifestyle, the action, and the camaraderie. This was the place that sparked my passion. By the end of my third summer at the White Dog, I had decided to pursue cooking as a career. I was a junior at Vanderbilt University, majoring in psychology (man, has that paid off in this business), with a concentration in philosophy, which I loved but didn't have the academic focus to study successfully. The volume of reading and paper writing nearly killed me. Again, the irony that I am now spending hours in front of a computer writing and editing is glaring, and I have found it to be even worse now.

The CIA

I had decided to apply to the Culinary Institute of America (CIA) and needed some experience on my resume, so I did a summer at the Opryland Hotel. I learned valuable knowledge in how to mass produce food. I acquired basic knife skills. I discovered what it means to be corporate in the restaurant industry. I found out early on that I really liked small-scale operations. I am sure this shaped me in other less obvious ways, I just haven't figured out what they are. I had my last summer on Nantucket after my job at the Opryland Hotel. The job lasted until Thanksgiving, and it was the last one before I would have to enter real life. Off to CIA.

I could write a whole book on the glorious education I received at CIA; but, that has been done already by others—and, really well, I might add. However, I must confess that the majority of what I learned came from outside the classroom. I think the saying goes: "school is as good as what you put into it." There is no place where that is truer than at culinary school. If you go through the motions, you are missing out on a whole other dimension of knowledge that is available. Volunteer for everything, participate in clubs, and work at parties. If there is an opportunity to cook with a chef, take it. The CIA was a great education, which I truly enjoyed, and I went from struggling through four years for a degree at Vanderbilt to graduating at the top of my class at CIA. I think that speaks volumes about the importance of passion in what you are doing. How did it shape me though? In what direction did it push me?

I believe the most valuable thing I learned in school was the importance of professionalism in the kitchen coupled with an understanding of the degree of intensity in my work that is needed to be truly successful in this business. It also provided me with a high level of standards for the quality of ingredients I use, for how I use those ingredients, and for my actions in everyday kitchen life. Now that I look back on it, this two-year period at CIA established my expectation of what a chef should be. It did exactly what school should do. It didn't define my cooking style at all, but it allowed me to develop a foundation on which to build. I got an incredible education in how to build flavors. I learned the importance of the history of gastronomy and the need to understand the past in order to forge your own future. I was exposed to different types of cooking. I really learned about the different types of food and where food comes from. Interestingly though, I don't remember any discussion of local foods versus industrial foods. Granted, my training came before any of the major books exposing the downside to industrial farming were published, but you'd think that would have been a logical part of the discussion. The CIA is usually on the leading edge of trends and advancements in the culinary world. (I have learned during the writing of this book they have indeed started a course in sustainability.) The next step came while I was still in school. It happened during my internship at the Inn at Blackberry Farm.

Blackberry Farm

WOW! Just in case that wasn't clear, WOW! I was there from 1996 to 1997 when Blackberry Farm was really starting to make its mark, and that was the single most impressive place I have ever worked. I took two things away from that experience: excellent customer service is essential, and using local ingredients is invaluable. This was my first real face-to-face encounter with using local food or the first time I worked in a restaurant that emphasized the use of local food. The best way to describe their service and the reputation that has driven many people their way is that they have an amazing ability to know what you want before you do. This, of course, is the key to good service, but I have never seen it executed with the ability that you find at Blackberry Farm. If you are thinking you might, *potentially*, have an itch, they will be there to scratch it. You will never see them, and the need will be completely satisfied before you've had time to identify it. It's like Southern hospitality meets Michelin stars at a laid-back hippie commune. Granted, this was a few years ago so it might have a slightly different atmosphere now, but I doubt it, especially with the comments I get from people in my own restaurant who have recently eaten there. It definitely showed me the type of service I wanted to emulate: passionate, intense, and detail-oriented while still holding on to individual personalities.

John Fleer was probably the chef closest to a mentor that I had; although I believe a mentor is someone you can turn to for advice and guidance repeatedly, and I didn't quite work with him long enough for that. He was pioneering Foothills cuisine and gave me my first experience with vegetables fresh from the garden, bacon and ham from locally raised pigs (which also happened to be from Allan Benton's smokehouse; not too shabby for a first taste), and local trout. I didn't realize the significance at the time; but, looking back, I recognize the importance of sourcing food from around the area. Even though Alice Waters had been doing it in California for years, it was really just starting to work its way throughout the country.

One memory, in particular, stands out. The AM sous at the time, Matt Rosencrantz, had forgotten to order the country ham for service for the next morning. He came to me and said, "Are you ready to go see where the bacon and ham come from?" In reality it was probably more like "Shit! I forgot to order the F***ing ham! Finish up and get your ass in the car. We're going to pick it up!" It wasn't really a choice as much as it was a directive, but I was there to learn and would basically do anything they asked. So we hopped in his car and drove about an hour to Madisonville, Tenn. It was like pulling up to the crossroads to make a deal with the devil. That is how good Allan's products are, and I've heard cooks say they would make that deal for some of his bacon. It was really the smokehouse in the middle of nowhere that helped conjure that imagery. You walked in to see these fabulous smoke rings on the walls and rows of curing country hams. Actually, it was more like pork heaven. I remember thinking on the way back that it was cool to be able to jump in a car and go pick up your product straight from the source. I wondered why more people didn't do that.

Back in Nashville

After graduating from CIA I returned to Nashville. I had some pretty big aspirations coming out of culinary school. I had graduated at the top of my class, had gotten lost in all things food, and was going to be somebody. However, I had decided to move to Nashville, not exactly the culinary mecca. I had gotten married right after culinary school and because my Southern wife had tolerated two years of snowdrifts while I was at CIA, I figured (that is, was told) it was her turn to finish her education and start her chosen career—so back to

Vanderbilt, back to Nashville. I knew there weren't going to be a lot of options, but I figured there would at least be a couple of restaurants where I could get some good experience and then we would move to a city with a little more culinary opportunity. Many years later I am still here.

I think I got lucky in my timing. The restaurant community in Nashville was pretty small when I first got into it. It was dominated by chains (an unfortunate fact that has not changed) with a spattering of independent restaurants (this, fortunately, has changed for the better). My first job out of school was at a start-up opened by a couple of Vanderbilt grads a few years older than I. I found out about the place through mutual friends and applied for the sous chef job. After all, I was a bad-ass CIA graduate. I was absolutely convinced I could manage a kitchen full of cooks. Oops. I was drilled for the first three months I was there. In hindsight, I can't believe I didn't get fired. Maybe my work ethic helped me keep my job because I think I worked 100 hours a week during those three months. I learned fast though, and quickly earned my chops and their respect. That place evolved into more of a bar than a restaurant, and I moved on after a year.

I do remember a conversation with one cook who had worked in every restaurant in the city—for reasons I soon understood, because he ended up being the first cook I ever fired. We were talking about the state of Nashville's culinary status. He said we were at the start of a culinary revolution in Nashville. In five years this place was going to be a food city. I was young and thought he was right. Actually, he was, almost; but, it took closer to ten years. We are still pretty unnoticed on the national level, which, with the talent of chefs in this city, is pretty astonishing.

I moved on to a corporate steakhouse next, realizing pretty quickly that it was not for me. But I hung on because, at the time, I thought I was leaving town when my wife finished school. I really learned how to manage a kitchen there. When a corporate office sets the pay rates it really limits the caliber of employee you can attract. I had a rag-tag bunch, and any day I didn't have to cover a no-show, break up a fight, bust somebody chugging booze or hitting a joint was a good day. I made a lot of mistakes and learned from them. I realized that I wanted to be in kitchens that allowed for creative exploration. I wanted to be in a kitchen with people who cooked with passion, not just for a paycheck. During this time, I played with the idea of opening a restaurant. It was my long-term goal, and when an opportunity presented itself, I followed it. I had already lost complete interest in the current restaurant and was fed up with the bullshit of the corporate world—broken promises, bonuses canceled for no reason. It basically sucked. I was tired of babysitting the cooks and ended up getting fired. Then the restaurant opportunity I followed fell through.

Eventually, I picked up at another restaurant in town called The Midtown Café as a cook and took over as chef pretty quickly. I think I was there about a year and a half. Business was pretty spotty. The place had been open for a while and never changed. I tried to change the menu, but was met with considerable resistance. There was little creative freedom, and most of the time I was boxed in by what they wanted me to do. The food in Nashville in the more upscale restaurants at that time was mostly Asian or Asian Fusion. I played in both styles, but never really got hooked. During my stint here I started to work again on opening a restaurant. This time I came as close as lease negotiations and some preliminary drawings. That deal didn't work out, but I had come to terms with the fact that I was in Nashville for the long haul. The other glorious part of my time at this restaurant was a chance to work with some local produce. It was very sporadic, and I didn't really pursue it aggressively, but it was there. More importantly, it tasted good.

I spent a very short period at one other restaurant during that time. I was devoted to opening my own place and had exhausted our savings, so I picked up one more job to tide me over until I succeeded in getting my place open. I had run a number of kitchens by now, and they all used the same products from the same people. Pick up the phone and make your order. I started to question why I followed this format. Was this the only option? Was stocking your kitchen solely about the lowest food cost and the bottom line?

FLYING SOLO

In 2003 I drove by the building that would become *tāyst*. It was around the middle of August. I had been working on opening a restaurant for a while so I pretty much had the business plan finished. I had been through a couple of potential partners and some negotiations for places I am glad I didn't get. So with a few tweaks to the plan, a small amount of money raised, and a new partner we signed the lease in October and opened in February 2004. It was a quick turn-around; but, I'm driven, and when I focus on a task, I get it done. I might add that we had to convert the building into a restaurant, as it was not one previously. Most people told me it couldn't be done, which only fueled my determination to make it happen.

After all this time in the business, this was the first restaurant in which I had ever been allowed to cook my own food. The first menu was definitely straight comfort food. I still used the same products from the same suppliers, and my menu was not really that different from what I had done in the restaurants where I had worked previously. Except for the fact that we used absolutely no Asian flavors whatsoever, we were just another independent restaurant in Nashville. Then I started to play. I started experimenting with "space food." I started really allowing my personality to pour into my dishes. I took it so far as trying to be weird for the sake of being weird. This was great for learning, not so good for business. I had pushed the boundaries too far and needed to rein myself back in. It is a business, and I needed to cook in a way that would fill the seats. At *tāyst* that came to be a blend of upscale and uncomplicated. We try to find subtle ways to get funky, but it's never over the top. I think the best way to describe it is having one foot firmly planted on each side of the line.

Standing Out and Setting Myself Apart

Something else developed during these years. I started to create first and think about functionality second. From the beginning we made everything to order. Initially, that decision was based on space—we didn't have room for a steam table. After a while, it was out of a sense of pride. We had this little neighborhood joint with anywhere from three to five cooks in the kitchen (including myself and the sous chef), and we made every dish fresh for an eighty-five-seat restaurant. That began to morph into making *everything* from scratch. We bought nothing premade. As our farmer connections increased, our processed food decreased. We made our own pasta. We made our own bread. We had always done desserts, but we stopped buying chocolate molds and other accessories. When we came up with a dish, it was definitely a "no fear" approach. In fact, my former sous used to joke about the fact that his purpose, besides running the kitchen while I was not there, was to keep my ideas in cheque. We have gone through many a cook because dishes were too hard to pull off during service. As far as I am concerned if you're good, you figure out a way to get it done. Difficulty should never interfere with the creative process. I think that can really be applied to just about every aspect of life. Why keep from experiencing something because it is hard? Experiencing failure is the key to success. If you have never failed at something, you can never know how success truly feels or what it will take to get there.

Throughout this time I continued reading all the food memoirs that were available. I didn't really read cookbooks; but I enjoyed the books that told restaurant stories, such as *Kitchen Confidential* by Anthony Bourdain, and *Letters to a Young Chef* by Daniel Boulud. My one big regret in my culinary career is that I never really took off and worked with a super famous chef at an exclusive restaurant. There was no French Laundry or El Bulli or L'Espalier. I didn't go to Europe and work in any Michelin starred restaurants. I didn't follow the typical path of the successful chef. However, missing this experience is a large part of the reason I am where I am today. This lack of tutelage in a rigid system allowed me to forge my own path and develop a style that is uniquely mine—that really encompasses all aspects of my evolution as a chef. For management, food, and service I had no real-life model to follow. At the time I was pushing my own boundaries I discovered some books that changed my views on how we grow our food: *Fast Food Nation*, *The Omnivore's Dilemma*, and *The Devil's Kitchen*. I was shown the light! Okay, it wasn't quite that dramatic, but it made me start to question even more where we sourced our foods. Marco Pierre White's book *The Devil in the Kitchen* doesn't offer much that fits this evolving philosophy; but there is one statement he made that rings true: "Great chefs respect nature."

Even before these books told us to do so, I had started using local farmers. But these books are not telling us to do something new. They are pointing out the negative aspects of the path we chose when we tried to modernize eating. They are showing us what is behind the million-dollar marketing plans. They are trying to remind us of where food comes from and what it takes to get it into the kitchen. With that basic principle in mind I was hitting the markets and meeting farmers. I was finding ways to incorporate those principles into the restaurant. I was working on building relationships. When we opened, I offered a menu that would change completely with each season. When I changed to the spring menu for the first time, it really freaked people out. There were a couple dishes people absolutely loved that were coming off the menu, and they couldn't believe it. I sat through not one, not two, but three different verbal lashings on how I was crazy to change my menu. I was told the dishes were outstanding and I was going to lose business if I let them go. I was given suggestions for how to keep them on the menu and still have a seasonal menu on the side. The trouble was, this was no different than some other menus in town, and with my overwhelming desire to be unique, that would never fly. Besides, why would it make sense to offer something like a cream sauce in 100-degree weather or promise berries that aren't ripe in December? My discoveries of local food and sustainability also prevented me from continuing some of these dishes. I was starting to make enough connections, to build enough relationships, to truly supply the restaurant with better tasting local food that, I was learning, had secondary benefits.

Being familiar with what Alice Waters was doing in California, I knew there was a growing underground movement toward popularizing local/organic food, though I didn't understand why. I engrossed myself in reading all the books in this genre. I wanted to know how everything was grown and what happened to the environment around it. I started realizing the true importance of buying locally grown food. Up to this point I had been doing it because the local produce had more flavor, but I was also learning the environmental effects are just as important. I realized that, at the rate we are destroying our soil, my grandchildren could potentially be forced to eat nothing but hothouse genetically modified organism (GMO) products. This became a hot issue for me, and one I'll explore in more detail in the following chapters. The point is I determined I needed to double my efforts to source local products.

Carving a Path

I began to really connect with some local farmers like Farmer Dave. I had used a few farmers over the years, but it was really hard to find local farmers. So, with religious fervor, I started hitting every farmers' market I could find. The downtown market in Nashville happens to be one of the only ones in the country open almost every day of the year. At the time, this market housed only a few product stalls, but filled a need as the other stalls were more like brokers or middlemen. Like the wine makers in Europe who buy grapes from small local growers and combine them to make wine to sell (negociants), these guys bought from local farmers and sold those products at the market. They also brought in industrial produce, so I learned I needed to talk to these guys and ask questions about where things were grown, how they were grown, etc. Eventually, I found other markets that were "producer only" markets; they were just beginning: These markets offered nothing but local food sold by the farmer who grew it. This is where I really got my education. I learned what the farmers did to rejuvenate their soil. I learned that the majority of small regional farmers followed organic practices even though they weren't certified. I started to find meat, dairy, and eggs from local sources. I began to develop relationships with these farmers. As they came to know me they realized I was passionate about what they were doing and wanted to share that with more people. My reputation and my mission were spreading throughout the farming community, and farmers who were just starting out began calling me. This created an opportunity for me to make special requests for them to grow things currently missing from the market. That was, and still is at this time, a huge step forward. It also solidifies the comment by Ferdinand Metz, that I had a real opportunity to shape the variety of food being grown in the region. Why is that important? Well, if we can ensure a good variety among the farmers, we can reduce the oversaturated marketplace and ensure all farmers' success. We are in the infancy of re-regionalizing our food system and we need farmers. If all our farmers are growing exactly the same products, then we will eventually lose some to competition; that's basic capitalism. If we truly are working toward a sustainable food system, we need to be increasing the number of farms.

A well-known fact, and a result of the post–World War II industrialization of the food industry, is that we have managed to completely separate ourselves from those who grow our food. This post-World War hypothesis is the generally accepted time frame for the shift in our food supply because it coincides with the integration of fertilizers and pesticides into modern agriculture, the steadily increasing farm subsidies, and basic technological advances. Think about that result. One of the most important things we require for our survival is food; ironically, we have come to no longer value our relationship with the growers or even remember they exist. The biggest dilemma we in the kitchen face, and one the next generation of chefs will continue to face, is rebuilding the relationship between the farmer and the consumer, in this case, the chef. Over the last couple of years Nashville has been successful in bringing these groups together. The response at these meetings has always been the same. The farmers want us to tell them what to grow, and the chefs want the farmers to show up with products for them to cook. It's like we are on opposite ends of a bridge, a bridge we built ourselves, and we don't know how to meet in the middle. I do think with each growing season we are closing the gap, but we still have a long way to go. There is also an underlying sense of warranted skepticism on both sides of the table. I think both sides have been burned at one time or another by expectations that were not met.

The goal for my restaurant was now clear: We would seek ways to rely on local sources for our food—as much as possible, as often as possible. I knew it would cost more, especially with meat; but I would not let cost be a deterrent. I wanted to find a way to emulate what I had seen at Blackberry Farm. In hindsight, I realized I had grown up with this style on Nantucket—a style I believed was the morally and socially responsible way to operate a business.

My food changed the more I sourced locally, but not in the ways you might imagine. Nashville is a funny town when it comes to food. We are a food town, but you have to come and eat here to know that. We have had an amazing boom of restaurants in the last five years. Are we New York or Chicago? No, but as far as a percentage of great restaurants per capita we are doing pretty well. The tastes of our town are unique, as they are in every town. I believe, to be successful in Nashville, you have to have a menu that balances gourmet and progressive with a touch of down-home meat and potatoes. We are also in a hotbed of chain restaurants. Like many other cities, we are in a constant battle against big budgets and million-dollar McMansion-style restaurants that have very large marketing machines behind them. In fact, *tāyst* is part of an organization called the Nashville Originals whose sole purpose is the success of the independent restaurants in Nashville. If I want to celebrate the local farmers and show them off to people, I need to be open, because, as I've stated before, the financial aspects of running a restaurant are significant and have to be considered. Without butts in the seats you won't be open for long. My food had to become more focused. I always cooked seasonally, but realized that the seasons didn't stop and start—they rolled. My menu started to reflect that roll. It became totally reliant on Mother Nature. We have cooked through drought and endless rain, bounty and slim pickin's. It still amazes me that I have been cooking for nearly twenty years and the weather just recently became a factor in my food. Also, my dishes became simpler because my product was so good on its own that I had to manipulate it less in order to get good flavors into the dish. As it turns out, the pure, unadulterated goodness of the ingredients was all I needed. All this is crazy talk, I know. But this is the way everybody should cook. The reality is, they don't. Is it changing? Yes. Farm-to-table is the hot trend right now, so you're seeing it across the country, from casual to fancy establishments. But for the most part, the majority of the food industry is not running their kitchens like this.

I think my playful side came out even more and found a place to run free as I made this transition. The dishes we were producing were a direct reflection of my personality. My cooking style really began to echo the passion growing in me for where my food came from and for the people who grew it. I had found my style, my voice, my future.

This chapter was very beneficial for me—putting this part of my journey on paper. It is wise to contemplate and reflect on how you got to where you are. I think it allows you to have a better idea of where you are heading, which, in turn, will help you focus more on the path ahead. I know what I want my food to be. I know what I want to say through my existing restaurant and future restaurants. My style is personal. It is playful. It is built on relationships and loyalty. It is built on community.

Chapter Three
Local and Sustainable

Locally produced food tastes better. It is the primary reason to source your food this way and to create a menu following the seasons. It is flat out better on the palate. For this reason, if for no other, the drive to buy local should be in every cook working in every kitchen across the country. If you work in a restaurant that doesn't buy local, ask your chef why not. Ask your owner why not. If it is because they don't know where to find local products, go out on your own and find the markets selling them. According to the USDA, the number of farmers' markets in our country has tripled in the last few years, and the ease in locating them is increasing as well. Since the USDA began to track farmers' markets in 1994, the number has grown by nearly 4,000 across the country, and the total number of markets in 2009 was 5,274 nationwide. A national directory of farmers' markets is available at http://www.ams.usda.gov/farmersmarkets.[6] If there is no market in your area, it is likely you will find a little produce store or a healthy food/whole foods market. The people who work in these places should be able to connect you with some farmers. If they are unaware of any local sourcing, then get online and search for local farms. Most state agricultural departments have a website with their state's farms and products listed. One of the purposes of the state branch of the USDA is to promote local and state products. There are also groups like the *Chefs Collaborative* whose purpose is to promote a sustainable food system. They, too, can link you with local farmers. Farmers are a close-knit community. You only need to meet one or two to have the whole network open to you. The other benefit of selecting your own farmers is that you will begin to develop relationships with the people who grow your food.

This relationship is a significant, if not primary, benefit of buying locally. Your relationships will allow you to become more connected to the land. This bond, this understanding, will be reflected in your food. Your guests will see the newfound "love" in your dishes. The respect you have for the food that comes through the kitchen door will increase exponentially. No longer will a pan of strawberries going bad bother you simply for the cost. (Not that it should be allowed to go bad anyway; but let's face it, it's busy and things slip through the cracks.) The difference is, when you physically see the land where the strawberries grew, and know the farmer who planted, weeded, picked, and maybe even delivered them, you will not let their work go to waste. Before you know it, you find yourself drying and canning what you can't immediately use in order to preserve the product. Suddenly you have flavors available in the winter when local growth is slow—flavors that were produced from food that was picked at the height of the season when it has the most taste, is at its cheapest, and might have gone bad as excess. By understanding the importance of the bond with my farmers, I came to realize the importance of having a relationship with all my purveyors. My farmers have become my friends, and dealing with them has become one of the most enjoyable aspects of being a chef.

Another objection you might encounter from your chef, or more likely your owner, is cost. If they say they don't source locally because of the expense involved, you need to pick up some local tomatoes or corn or lettuce and show them the difference. There will not only be a noticeable contrast in flavor, but it will have a much better quality and a longer shelf life. With this improved quality you will get increased yield as well as extended usage out of fresh local product. For example, take an industrial tomato out of Chile or some other distant place. It's picked unripe in order to extend its life so it can make it to the market, which, in this case, is a grocery store. This tomato will be gassed during travel so when it gets to your door it is a beautiful, perfectly red tomato. Fresh vegetables begin to produce a gas called ethylene after being picked. According to the Ethylene Control website, ethylene causes fruits to ripen and decay, and causes wilting in vegetables and floral products. "Controlling ethylene gas after picking will extend the life cycle of your commodity—allowing them to be held for a much a longer period of time."[7] After scientists were able to construct controlled environments, they were able to utilize man-made ethylene to control the ripening process. The problem with this is that the tomato will be barren of any flavor and, when you cut into it, the core will probably still be white. You will have to discard a large portion of this tomato because it is inedible (or at least will taste like cardboard). Whatever plans you have for that tomato will require more manipulation and stronger seasonings to create a flavorful dish. All these factors increase the cost of your tomato in the end. The opposite is true for a local, seasonal tomato. All that is necessary is to pick it, wash it, add a pinch of salt, and eat it. Ultimately, you will find the cost of the decreased yield—not getting the full and best use of your industrial product—makes the initial cost difference of your local produce seem less problematic. If enough people start buying seasonally and locally, the cost of production will eventually come down. In my experience, the cost difference of produce is already minimal at best.

When you consider the increasing cost of industrial foods resulting from, among other factors, the inevitable rise in the cost of fossil fuels, you'll find the claim of greater cost-effectiveness to be less and less true. The fact is, food prices around the world are rising. The recently released Food and Agriculture Organization (FAO) of the United Nations 2010 food price index indicates that, "compared to 2002–2004, commodity food prices sharply increased, especially those of sugars and fats. The new index is higher than in 2008 when people throughout the world rioted in protest. It is also at the highest level recorded since the index began in 1990."[8] (See Table 1 in Appendix A.) It is the simple principle of supply and demand. The decrease in croplands, increase in weather events, and elevated oil prices are all contributing factors in failing supplies, which are driving up prices. So, when you consider the cost savings of buying locally, from a community perspective, and couple that with having less waste and pollution, decreased fossil fuel usage, and less packaging, the balance sheet speaks for itself.

WHY BUY LOCAL?

So, now you may ask: What are the other reasons to buy local, and what does it have to do with being green and sustainable? I'll explain it this way. I like to accumulate knowledge, specifically food-related knowledge. In my drive for information, I have also passed my discoveries on to everyone who works for me in order to ensure they have the same passion for dining green that I do. I can't require them to go home and read, but I can suggest some documentaries that successfully represent some of the reasons for my operational overhaul. I've started accumulating a DVD library, and my staff is strongly encouraged to watch these documentaries. One of these films is called "How to Save the World: One Man, One Cow, One Planet." It explores the recent surge of biodynamic farming in India, exploring the impact of the green revolution and the positive effects of sustainable farming. The following is a statement from that film that really drives home the need for an internal evaluation of *our* nation's food supply:

> A sustainable farm is a regenerative and living organism that maintains its productivity and usefulness to society indefinitely. It is resource conserving, socially supportive, commercially competent, and environmentally sound.[9]

Basically, this is the definition of a sustainable farm. It means a farm that takes care of itself will be successful in producing not just for the farmers, but the community. Most importantly, it will have a positive, regenerative effect on the environment instead of leaving the Earth depleted. Whether certified organic or biodynamic, or just a small farmer using sensible and responsible growing practices, the sustainable farm will continue to be productive forever. This is not true for conventional or industrial farming. An industrial farm dealing with commodity crops—probably genetically modified—is incapable of continually producing for generations to come. Genetically modified organism (GMO) crops must be purchased each year. Some seed companies have inserted a terminator gene into their product that causes the plant to commit suicide after one fruiting.

Some GE [Genetically Engineered] seeds are engineered so that plants cannot reproduce seeds. In many parts of the world, saving seeds from season to season is the only way farmers are able to survive and continue growing food. However, with GE technology, seeds can be sterile, forcing farmers to rely on seed companies for their livelihood, an expense they may not be able to bear.[10]

That fact, in itself, makes a farm commercially incompetent. I will include this caveat: At the recent International Foodservice Sustainability Symposium, Dr. Roger Beachy, one of the inventors of GE seeds, stated that at the current time no "terminator genes" were in use anywhere in the world.

Regardless of whether they are in use or not, what successful business model is founded on making the same initial investment over and over again when it should be a renewable asset? What would make a business investor want to sign up for that? The only benefit is in the profits for the people holding the seed patent. In the restaurant business it would be like buying new pans after they are used one time to produce a dish. Think about that in terms of your household. Would you buy new light fixtures every time a light bulb burned out, instead of simply replacing the bulb? The commercial incompetency is also evidenced in the necessity for government subsidies to support the industrial farms incapable of making a profit without it. Or is it that the subsidies changed the way farms were worked, forcing their dependency on industrial practices in order to get the funds? Chicken or the egg conundrum, anyone?

56

TO SUBSIDIZE OR NOT TO SUBSIDIZE

I don't want to get into a debate regarding farm subsidies; yet we need to touch on it because it absolutely affects the ability to buy locally. I am not for the instant and absolute abolishment of farm subsidies. You'll see, as with most issues regarding restructuring our food system, there are no easy answers. I asked my farmers about their feelings on subsidies, none of whom receive any subsidies, by the way. Their response is similar to that of subsidy supporters: To eliminate subsidies would mean the farms under that umbrella of support would go bankrupt, and the world would starve. They're right. Even as a layman (not an economist, scientist, farmer, or politician), I see two possible answers as a solution toward the removal of farm subsidies.

The first possibility is to slowly shift the criteria for subsidies from farms growing one or two commodity crops to farms growing a wide range of food. Through a polyculture form of farming these farms could produce more nutrients per acre and replenish the health of the soil. And, if not polyculture farming, at least a significant variety and rotation of product could ensure natural soil replenishment. Farmers who show significant soil improvement can gain extra incentives. Ideally, the system would evolve into a replenishing farm system, and the farmers would be making a profit. Part of this sustainable farm model is that as it becomes environmentally sustainable it will also become financially sustainable. The addition of subsidies to these sustainable farm models can positively affect the ability of these farms to offer their products to a larger portion of the country by being able to decrease prices. At this moment the cost of much of this produce is too high for many consumers. This is particularly true for those in food deserts, or areas within urban centers in which access to "real" food is limited and the percentage of obese, malnourished people is higher. The more people buying from these farmers, the better their chances for being profitable; this greatly improves the chances for increasing the number of farmers. Besides, isn't cheap food exactly what the current subsidies accomplish? In fact, it is the main reason our food is deceptively cheap.

Once these renovated farms move toward becoming profitable, subsidies could be decreased and those resources moved to investments in future farms or, better yet, in young start-up farmers. According to Michael Pollan, the average age of farmers in this country is 55.[11] To break the stats down even further, the percentage of U.S. farmers 65 and older in 1978 was 16.6%, in 2002 it was 26.2%. Alternatively, the percentage of farmers under 35 in 1982 was 15.9% and in 2002 it was 5.8%. The total population of farmers makes up only 1% of the 315 million people in our country.[12] When you combine the age of these farmers with the fact that the knowledge needed to farm successfully is disappearing with each generation of farmers lost, you have a recipe for disaster, even more than that created by the chemical destruction of our soil. All the wonders of genetic modification can't make seeds plant and harvest themselves. Let alone decide when the time is right to do so. Think about that. Granted, this is a worst case scenario, but it is something to be considered carefully.

The second option for removing subsidies and revamping the food system, and a major reason to buy local, is to eliminate the legality of seed patenting, and, ultimately, removing the use of GMO seeds for food altogether. The largest receivers of subsidies are corporate farms that plant genetically engineered corn and soybeans. According to the

Environmental Working Group, the top 20% of farms received 80% of the subsidies.[13] Though this may not be a viable option at the moment, what potentially does have a chance is labeling the use of GMO foods in our country. We are one of the only countries in the world that does not force food companies to reveal the use of the GMOs on the label. Seventy percent of processed foods in American supermarkets now contain genetically modified ingredients.[14] Contacting your local congressman and voting can make a difference in getting this practice legislated. The profit margin of these food companies is slim. Even a slight change in their revenue would force them to adapt. This labeling information would at least give us a chance to choose what we are putting into our bodies; even more importantly, our children's bodies. To quote the local food movement's mantra, this labeling information would truly allow us to "vote with our dollar."

DEFINING THE PROBLEM

By eliminating the legality of seed patenting, and eventually GMOs, we eliminate a key link in the chain of the industrial food system. When we cannot use patented seeds altered to flourish in the low-labor, high-chemical, and pesticide-laden industrial environment, the current subsidy system is no longer functional. If you look at the seed controllers' argument for the patent, they claim they have changed the makeup of the genes within the seed; therefore, they own the seed itself. The logical extensions of this argument take us into some frightening territory—particularly if you accept the words of Jean Anthelme Brillat-Savarin: "Tell me what you eat and I will tell you who you are." It is dangerous for corporations to be allowed to claim ownership of such fundamental parts of our existence. The philosophical and ethical discussion that follows brings up issues of the control of life itself. A scary discussion.

Maybe the scariest part of the discussion is that I am just scratching the surface of some of the components of the current food system. There are a number of resources out there for educating yourself further on the issues surrounding the state of the food system, such as *The Omnivore's Dilemma* by Michael Pollan, *Fast Food Nation* by Eric Schlosser, or *Food Matters* by Mark Bittman. (A larger list is provided in the appendix.) However, if your regional newspaper is anything like ours, you don't have to go any further than it to find a plethora of featured food articles covering these issues. The titles will read something like this: *Small Farmers Being Crushed—Forced to Sell to Developers Due to Loss of Profitability; Hundreds Nationwide Sick with Salmonella* [or E. coli, or some other food-borne illness]. Remember this: After eating contaminated food, people can develop anything from a short, mild illness (often mistakenly referred to as "food poisoning") to life-threatening diseases. The Centers for Disease Control and Prevention (CDC) estimates that 76 million, or one quarter of, Americans get sick from what they eat. More than 300,000 are hospitalized, and 5,000 people die from food-borne illnesses each year.[15] Some other headlines recently proclaimed, *U.S. Officially Fattest Country in World* and *Farmers Struggle to Put Food on Table.* That last one is particularly disturbing. Now take a look at the positive reporting on food-related issues. *New Farmers' Market on Saturdays at Corner of Hope and Community. Local Chef Goes Green* (couldn't help it). *Community Garden Started in Impoverished Urban Food Desert.* (You would be amazed at how many food deserts there are in our metropolitan areas.) If you read all those articles, you'll notice a unique difference—the sheer difference in scope. The negative articles are overwhelmingly on a national level, and, in contrast, the positive ones are limited to small victories by local communities.

The overall message is fundamentally the same. The green revolution of the mid-twentieth century took the control of farming away from the farmers and put it in the hands of multinational corporations. The process of growing food was no longer a personal investment. It became more industrialized, more commodified, and more dependent on industrial refinements each year. We have reached a point where food production must rely on government subsidies to survive. The basic key to life has been patented into such restriction that what once offered a natural bounty of variety is now relegated to *no* choice. In the documentary "How to Save the World" an astonishing statistic was quoted:

> There were once 30,000 different types of rice grown in India. Now there are fifteen. That means the wonderful opportunities for creativity from cooks as well as the diversity between regions (foodsheds) will be quashed by the lack of variety in food.[16]

GENETICALLY MODIFIED

The same problem is happening in the corn industry in the United States and in Mexico as well. There are areas of Mexico that have never planted a GMO product, though corn harvested from some of their crops shows genetically modified material. A 2004 North American Free Trade Agreement (NAFTA) report showed "researchers found that some forms of genetically modified corn were present in Mexico and were being naturally spread by cross-pollination . . . Although it remains uncertain how the modified corn got into Mexican fields, the report concluded that the large-scale importation of U.S. corn was the likely cause."[17] The reason they were importing that corn is because it was cheaper for them to eat imported American corn than the corn they were growing. Seeds are a living thing, fighting for survival like all other living things. They have evolved over thousands of years, developing characteristics that allow them to self-propagate and flourish. It is impossible to rein in or control these aspects of nature. This means that when we attempt to do so and tamper with the natural order we end up with unanticipated, and usually undesirable, results.

I do believe, in the beginning, the scientists and companies involved in genetic modification truly intended for this to benefit humanity, for these advances to improve our ability to provide for the expanding population; however, that is no longer the case. The companies in control have been derailed from their original vision and are being driven by the almighty dollar. Although their publicly stated goals say otherwise, the evidence of this speaks too loudly to be denied. While they might claim to be held to a higher standard because of the nature of what they do, the fact remains they are in business to make a profit. While this is true of companies of all sizes, the difference between big and small organizations is in the personal involvement in day-to-day operations. It's easy to lose sight of your purpose and focus on the task at hand, which, in the case of large corporate companies, is shareholder interests. It reminds me of sitting in the backyard watching my daughters play. They can be so easily distracted and diverted to another interest, requiring them to let go of something that, at one time, was so important they shed tears to keep it. This distraction results in a melted popsicle or escaped fireflies. Obviously as adults we are capable of focusing more firmly on the tasks in front of us, but we never lose that potential for distraction. Every "how to" business book tells you to write a business plan that is detailed, and to refer back to it often to ensure that you remain on the path that you laid out in the beginning. There has to be a reason for that. Our natural tendency to stray from our original path, perhaps? It is important for us to pause, reevaluate the state of affairs, identify where we went wrong, and fix it before those things we cherished slip away from us.

CONVENTIONAL VS. SUSTAINABLE FARMING

So, what really is the difference between conventional farming and sustainable farming? Conventional farming is also known as "industrial farming" or "modern agriculture." According to the USDA:

> Conventional farming systems vary from farm to farm and from country to country. However, they share many characteristics: rapid technological innovation; large capital investments in order to apply production and management technology; large-scale farms; single crops/row crops grown continuously over many seasons; uniform high-yield hybrid crops; extensive use of pesticides, fertilizers, and external energy inputs; high labor efficiency; and dependency on agribusiness. In

63

the case of livestock, most production comes from confined, concentrated systems.[18]

"Uniform high-yield hybrid crops" means farming with GMO seeds (which need chemicals and fertilizers in order to be productive), though it is beyond me how it can be considered so. Truthfully, isn't this the opposite of what it really means to farm? It is tragic that completely manipulated, "juiced" food is considered conventional. I think of the major controversies surrounding steroid use in professional sports. Is this not precisely what we are doing to our food? If this aspect of the food world got even half the coverage given to the sports world, the public outcry would be overwhelming. Apply this philosophy to the restaurant landscape (it's already being done, by the way), and it raises the question of whether that can be considered cooking. If the product you serve is processed and manipulated to the point of uniformity, are you still cooking? Is it still food?

The Problem with Conventional Farming

One of my goals is to show a basic correlation between the need to source locally and how that affects our long-term need for food sources, period. Ongoing research, and even the USDA resources, shows that conventional farming is harmful to the soil. Yet, even as we encounter pesticide-resistant bugs and serious soil destruction we respond with increased uses of the same techniques and invest in growing crops without soil. Eventually we will run out of productive soil with which to farm. It is probably not going to happen in my lifetime; but, at the rate we are going, we will reach a point in my children's lives when we will not easily find places to source food. If we don't change the way in which we farm, they won't have very

64

many options. If the worst happens, they will have no options at all.

Basically, a conventional farm plants the same crops year in and year out in the same soil. Some of them will alternate between two types of crops; but, for the most part, they use a monoculture style of farming. The natural effect of this repetitive planting is a stripping of the nutrients in the soil. Historically this is one of the main reasons crops were varied and rotated. In order to counter this nutrient loss, fertilizers are used to reintroduce those stripped nutrients into the soil. These fertilizers become part of the soil destruction. These synthetic nutrients eventually find their way into the groundwater. The groundwater runs into streams, which run into rivers, which run into the ocean. This causes something called algal bloom.

Here is a great description of the effects of algal bloom: "When large amounts of nitrogen collect in a water body, eutrophication can result. This is an accumulation of excess nutrients which causes an algae bloom. The algae rapidly deplete all of the oxygen in the water, making it unlivable for fish and other aquatic organisms."[19] What is amazing is how well known this problem is, and yet proponents still argue that chemical farming is a good thing. If the runoff prevents life in one area, chances are good that it is affecting life in other areas we might not see. What does it take to keep an issue this large relatively quiet? Why doesn't this raise questions on a larger public scale as to how this type of farming is affecting our environment? The irony of using these fertilizers is that we have had to alter the way we farm in order to accommodate the invention of the fertilizers. Essentially, they were not invented out of necessity.

This soil that is constantly bombarded each year with unnatural nutrients is also bombarded with pesticides used to protect the plants. Plants were once grown from saved seeds that built up immunities to most of the pests and environment around them, in combination with crop rotation and companion planting. These seeds have been swapped for "super seeds" that are modified to resist all pesticides in order to allow for easier farming. By engineering these plants, weeds and bugs alike can be killed with one spraying. In layman's terms, it is basically like Concentrated Animal Feeding Operations (CAFOs)—in which antibiotics are given to cows in close confinement in order to ward off bacterial infections. By the same token, plants are given pesticides to fight off threatening insects and pests. Now we are seeing resistant super-weeds that have evolved in order to withstand the pesticides much like super bacteria have evolved thanks to the overload of antibiotics used in CAFOs. So we are using more pesticides to kill those and falling into a vicious cycle of chemical reliance.

Eventually the pesticides follow the same path to contaminating the watershed as the fertilizers. But they have a secondary effect. They kill not only the pests, but, in tandem with the fertilizer, destroy the other living matter in the soil— the natural flora. The soil eventually loses its life, becoming hard and dry. Without the humus, or life, in the soil it loses its ability to hold moisture. Water runs more freely through it and erosion becomes an issue. Erosion causes a loss of soil, changes the environment for all inhabitants. It's like a one-two punch with a knockout blow. Elaine Ingham of the *Agroforestry E-journal* explains: "If the numbers of bacteria, fungi, protozoa, nematodes and arthropods are lower than they should be for a particular soil type, the soil's 'digestive system' doesn't work

66

properly. Decomposition will be low, nutrients will not be retained in the soil, and will not be cycled properly. Ultimately, nutrients will be lost through the groundwater or through erosion because organisms aren't present to hold the soil together."[20]

Energy is also a highly consumed resource for conventional farming. The fertilizers are petroleum-based and require large amounts of energy to be manufactured. Then fuel is needed to run the equipment for the planting, spraying, and harvesting. Basically, the more mechanized an operation becomes the more fuel it uses. Plus, the amount of fuel required to ship food to market is excessive and, only now, with the concern for global warming, is being considered in calculating the energy drain created by conventional farming. As leading food journalist Tom Philpott states, in conventional farming "our fresh produce in most regions of the country log between 1,500 and 2,000 miles on the road."[21] This means that the meat-and-three you have for lunch could potentially travel up to 6,000 miles. That's just lunch. It also doesn't take into account how much fuel went into producing the meat of that meat-and-three. Pollan stated in his March 2002 *New York Times Magazine* article, "This Steer's Life," that it takes almost 284 gallons of oil to get one cow to market. One barrel is 42 gallons and a drum is 55 gallons. When the cost of crude oil shoots up - over $100 again, it's more than your gas money that is affected. The energy use adds up quickly. (See Table 1 in Appendix A for a chart of food price changes.)

Finally, conventional farming in many third world countries requires workers to manually spread pesticides. In our country, modern agriculture has significantly decreased the need for labor, but the labor that is used, typically migrant workers, also encounters pesticide exposure. Supposedly there is no harm to humans, but that is hard to believe. The purpose of this product is to kill everything except the seeds, which are genetically modified to withstand the pesticides. While the green revolution is happening worldwide, not just in our community, the majority of the regulations we have in place for worker safety in the United States are not followed overseas or south of our borders, and sometimes not within our borders. The safety of farm workers must be taken into consideration. Even if you couldn't care less about the environmental effects or the manipulation of our food, the human element should be cause for alarm.

Global Considerations

When we talk about the environmental concerns connected with the growth of food we must consider the global impact. As we have seen in the results of conventional farming outlined previously, one effect causes another, and environments miles away can be hurt through local actions. For most third world countries, the attractiveness of conventional farming was found in the perceived ability to generate much more food per acre than is possible in organic farming, thus making their farms more productive and increasing their ability to provide for their families. This is true, provided they use GMO seeds, fertilizers, and pesticides. Sadly, many of the farmers following that path are finding out the harsh realities of crop failure, health issues, and serious debt. Most foreign farms are not covered by government subsidies. They are losing their land and fleeing to the slums of the cities. Generations of a sustainable existence are collapsing into farms that are unable to feed their families. If farmers can't feed their families, it begs the question: What is the next group they won't be able to feed?

Another aspect of growing concern stemming from farmers buying into the hype of industrial farming is deforestation. Farmers are cutting down areas of rain forests for the misguided goal of cashing in on the global grain and meat market. Deforestation has been on the radar of most people, even those not so environmentally conscious, for some time. To refresh the discussion, these are the major effects.

"The removal of trees without sufficient reforestation has resulted in damage to habitat, biodiversity loss, and aridity. Deforested regions often degrade into wasteland."[22] The path to that "wasteland" is quickened by erosion. Erosion happens faster through the use of chemicals such as pesticides and fertilizers in industrial farming. Eventually we have the chain reaction of loss of biodiversity and destruction of the living elements of that ecosystem.

You may speculate: Conventional farming must have some benefits. Why else would it have taken hold the way it has? The truth is there are benefits, and they are pretty simple. It takes much less labor in order to work the farm. It makes cheap food available for everyone. Although I think the cost-effective benefit is arguable since the existence of this food, in our country, is based on government subsidies. However, according to proponents of industrial agriculture, "industrial ag produces higher yields, and as global population grows, we're going to have to squeeze as much food as possible out of the earth, by any means necessary, to produce enough sustenance."[23] It makes sense on a practical level. If this method produces higher yields, then industrial farming is the key to feeding the 7 billion people throughout the world. It is really hard to complain about those benefits. However, the questions remain. For how long can we maintain this? And at what cost? Aren't we failing to feed the world right now, even with a significant amount of industrial agriculture being used? Obviously, my argument is somewhat biased and weighted in favor of sustainable farms. Also, as previously stated, I haven't done more than scratch the surface of the intricacies of conventional farming and its effects on the environment. Each individual issue related to conventional farming can be discussed and debated for days. I don't expect to convince everyone, nor do I believe we can do away with all industrial farms, immediately. I do hope, however, to get your interest piqued and prompt you to search for more information. I encourage you to start asking questions and challenge the status quo on where your food comes from and how it is grown. And, hopefully, this will lead you to considering how to operate your restaurant. This chapter is about local and sustainable food sources and it may seem as if I have strayed from that focus, but the understanding of how food is grown in the current system is paramount to fortifying your move to a local infrastructure.

The Benefits of Sustainable Farming

So, let's talk about the real benefit of sustainable farming. It is sustainable. Done. That was easy. Actually, I guess we should briefly talk about the different kinds of farming going on right now that produce sustainable food. Then we can look at the benefits that come from farming in this manner.

In the sustainable world there are two types of farming most commonly used and discussed: biodynamic farming and organic farming. Biodynamic farming is basically organic farming with a touch of hippie star-loving, or the melding of "a sophisticated understanding of ecological processes with a faith in the power of the moon, sun, planets, and other cosmic forces to influence crops."[24] The actual definition in its most simple terms is the process of producing food naturally without the use of synthetic chemical fertilizers and genetically modified organisms.[25] In recent years the government has become involved in the control and regulation of organic labeling. They define it this way:

> Organic food is produced by farmers who emphasize the use of renewable resources and the conservation of soil and water to enhance environmental quality for future generations. Organic meat, poultry, eggs, and dairy products come from animals that are given no antibiotics or growth hormones. Organic food is produced without using most conventional pesticides; fertilizers made with synthetic ingredients or sewage sludge; bioengineering; or ionizing radiation. Before a product can be labeled "organic," a Government-approved certifier inspects the farm where the food is grown to make sure the farmer is following all the rules necessary to meet USDA organic standards. Companies that handle or process organic food before it gets to your local supermarket or restaurant must be certified, too.[26]

Through biological controls, crop rotation, green manures, livestock variation and rotation, and other environmentally friendly techniques, organic farming is

71

essentially a return to the original means of farming used for generations before us. It is a path chosen by farmers who are embracing the demand for food produced not only in an environmentally friendly way but which tastes better and is more nutritious.

Biodynamic Agriculture was developed by Austrian scientist and philosopher Rudolf Steiner in the early 1900s. Biological cycles and "dynamic"—metaphysical or spiritual— aspects of the farm are employed in biodynamic farming with the goal of balancing physical and non-physical realms.[27] Biodynamic farmers pay attention to the stars as much as to the earth. By using a combination of all aspects of the world they believe they can grow better food more successfully. Some practices include rituals such as filling an empty cow horn with manure and burying it in a field to increase the fertile aspects of the field. The stirring of compost mixed with water in a certain fashion as well as the method with which it is distributed are examples of other biodynamic techniques.

Organic Agriculture is the other type of farming rarely discussed that I believe is vital for the true success of the "re-new-ed" food system. Considering the state of our agriculture today, I feel these farmers—the local farmers—are necessary for chefs, consumers like you and me, to survive. You hear about certified organic farmers, industrial farmers, and even biodynamic farmers; you especially hear about buying local. However, a large group of farmers comprising the bulk of that ability to buy local get lost; they are the ones who farm sustainably without certification. In advocating for these farmers, I realize I am contradicting myself when I push for organic and green certification; but I am okay with that for a few reasons. First and foremost, I have spent the time to develop a relationship with these folks. They are typically farmers with small operations, growing on a small amount of land. Many are just getting started, although that is not always the case. They do not have the means, the time, or the desire to go though the certification process with the government. However, they know their clients: their community supported agriculture (CSA) members and the chefs who buy directly from them.

They farm organically because it is important to them and they realize the benefits of this type of farming. As with my green certification, the purpose of an organic label or the certification of a farmer allows them to reach a broader base of consumers and validates them for new clients. Certification is an integral part of establishing the initial relationship with the consumer when that consumer is removed from direct interaction. I think this demonstrates the importance of developing a relationship with your farmer. I would have never found out how these local farmers treated their product and their land without asking questions and learning about their practices. I have met the majority of my farmers through the relationships I forged with other farmers, which is really the best stamp of certification.

The reality is a sustainable farm has the ability to produce forever. This really isn't a new concept. Farmers have worked the land this way for thousands of years. It has been only in the last sixty years that we are facing major issues with the future of our food supply, and the soil is at the root of this crisis. We are on the verge of causing irreparable harm to our farming soil, which has an immeasurable impact on our ability to continue producing food with any nutritional value, not to mention its importance to our ability to live on the earth. We are also, in this country, removing the available growing soil at an astonishing rate through urban development and sprawl.

The key to sustainable farming is its ability not only to conserve but to enhance the soil. The good news is sustainable farmers using practices that include cross planting, rotation, cover crops, and natural pest protection will naturally end up with better soil. If we stop spraying and saturating our land with chemicals and begin to use proper farm practices, the soil can be restored. The biodynamic revolution in India is a great example of how a country can change. The biodynamic farms there have shown an increase in their water table and a decrease in their water usage by as much as 50%.[28] This study was performed on farms that were once using conventional practices and have switched to biodynamic farming. Once again, their soil has the ability to produce nutritious food, resist droughts, and feed their families. Farming is still a business and farmers must make money to survive. Unfortunately, these practices have been billed as costly and time consuming. The truth is, the demand is there for this type of product and these farms can be profitable. However, it will mean work and creativity on their part to find the right market.

WHY MAKE THE CHANGE?

Earlier, I touched on the bridge developing between the farmer and the consumer. We are in the very early stages of seeing a shift of eating habits back to a local food–based diet. We're realizing that we are fat!!! Farmers are learning how to communicate with their market again and people are learning how to talk about "real" food again. I am fortunate to have fabulous sources for local food. It wasn't that easy for me to get there. It was especially difficult to find a good source for meats, particularly beef; but I was persistent in my efforts. One farm in particular took extreme persistence. My first organic, grass-fed start-to-finish, beef farmer, was a farm called West wind farms. They were a little chef-shy in the beginning, but eventually modified their production, however slightly, to incorporate my needs. It probably took six to eight months from the first time I discovered them at a farmers' market to get him to come around. I bought some samples of their steaks and loved them. At the next market I asked about getting larger restaurant-style cuts. They explained it was not something he typically provided, but promised they would cut some at the next processing. I waited, and around the time it was due I asked for my order. I was told, "Not yet, it will be ready in a few weeks." I waited again, and then asked for my order after the designated time, only to be disappointed. This was the way it went for a few months. I began to feel as though I was dealing with the "Soup Nazi." My guess is the farmers had been burned by chefs before and wanted to make sure I wasn't going to place an order and never pick it up. When I finally got my first order, we went through the meat in about three weeks. The farmer was a little surprised, to say the least. The second round took a little while as well, but since that time I've been receiving a delivery within days of my order every time. I was able to establish a relationship by showing them I was serious about using their product and that I could sustain my demand enough to make it worth the extra effort.

Profitability is a key part of this discussion. Affordability is equally as important, particularly from the consumer's point of view. It is true that, right now, the cost of local/organic food is higher and, carrot for carrot, meat for meat, the purchase price of organic/local food will typically be higher. However, when individuals evaluate it on the cost-benefit scale, most decide the quality and the benefits are well worth the expense. On the wholesale side the cost-benefit scale will show the same results. Right now the demand for local, sustainable product far outweighs the supply. Based solely on what we are seeing in CSA sales and farmers' markets, even in these hard economic times, people are still choosing to pay a higher price for food they know is healthy. On the local level these farms have real potential to be extremely profitable if they are willing to adapt to their market and take advantage of the demand.

On the other hand, the most important aspect of buying locally, in my opinion, is that every dollar you spend stays in your community. That money is put back into your schools, your health care, and your roads. It is not going through three middlemen on its way to some foreign land. It's staying right where you are and supporting your local businesses. A recent study showed nearly two-thirds of consumers surveyed are willing to frequent a company that supports local businesses and sustainable practices.[29]

Farming and food are an integral part of the survival of our species, and there is a fundamental connection between the land and the community that should not be ignored or undermined. While we are not going to de-globalize our economies or our business strategies, it does not mean we can't take a step back and reevaluate which businesses should operate on a global scale. We have certainly benefited from the globalization of the food industry in our opportunities for experiencing the flavors of other cultures. Replicating a dish from our travels or having a wider variety of dining options is valuable, and I would not want to take that away. It isn't a matter of having one to the exclusion of others. It's a matter of balance and wise choices. Food was traded globally for centuries before the industrial food revolution put us on the path we are on now. Perhaps the answer is an even stronger push for an emphasis on a local-based diet. If we cultivate an atmosphere or market in which local farmers can grow their food in a way that is environmentally friendly, the food travels less to get to the market, takes less energy to produce, requires less water, and provides an affordable and profitable option for farmers and consumers, we are naturally creating a sustainable food system. Then you can still feel good about leaving room on our grocery shelves for that global flavor—things like organic olive oil, crystallized ginger, organic soy sauce, and balsamic vinegar. Sustainable farming is growing on a global scale. On the occasions you look outside your foodshed for food, look for the sustainable options. This is an example of when the *Green* certification comes in handy.

When we look at buying from local and sustainable sources it can be an overwhelming vision. But once the change begins you will find it gets easier. You will find it will work if you practice the habit of deciding, when it is time to get veggies, that you will go to the market and get what is in season. Does this choice mean you can't get a tomato in December? YES. But it also means that first tomato of the season will taste so much better. It might be a trade-off, but one that has so many benefits in the long run. When I talk about benefits I am not just referring to the ones that directly affect you and your restaurant, but the secondary benefits of an improved community and environment as well. The best help we can give the world is to focus on buying sustainable.

Second tāyst

Chapter Four
Land-Based Proteins

There is a clearly discernable link between the use of local goods and the sustainability of our environment. It is a widely known fact that the average food travels 1,500 miles before it hits your plate, yet many people still don't make the connection with the impact this has on sustainable resources. A major selling point of the buy-local movement has been the decrease in miles your food travels to get to your door. However, that alone does not mean all local food is sustainable and all sustainable food is local. Sustainable options are growing, but sometimes what can be found locally isn't always the best choice. When we discuss sustainability, for the restaurant industry, it is important to consider its carbon footprint. But we must also look beyond the carbon impact to the other long-term effects, including the use of hormones, pollution from improper waste disposal, best practices in land use, and human health implications, to name a few. These are all current hot topics relevant to the overall environmental health, but I feel they can be left out of the greater environmental discussion which focuses so much on greenhouse gases and climate change.

From an agricultural point of view, this correlation between the health of the environment and the style of farming employed can be easily demonstrated by examining the differences between organic vegetables versus industrial commodity vegetable crops. Cattle, pigs, poultry, and fish have become traded commodities just like . . . OIL. I realize food imports/exports have global trade implications; but, even trying to think like an economist, I cannot look at food in the same framework as widgets. Maybe "commodification" is one of the underlying problems in the food system, one of the reasons we have been so easily removed from our connection with food.

Regardless of the reasons, we know that the current food system has many problems with no happy endings. We also know that the food system is complex, and the connection between our food growing practices and our environmental health runs much deeper than organic vegetables versus industrial vegetables. While we can use that as an example to gain a basic understanding of the environmental impact of growing food, we still have to recognize the facts. Within this complex structure, any imbalance causes ripple effects throughout the entire food system. All the varying means for producing, distributing, consuming, and removing food should be considered in the construction of a sustainable system. In fact, to compartmentalize the food groups for an environmental evaluation in such a way downplays and disguises the grand scale of the issues at hand. There are those in the local food movement (Pollan comes to mind) who claim it was this very failure to view our food sourcing and consumption in a holistic manner that has led to some of the problems plaguing our society—specifically our mounting health concerns.

That being said, it is actually necessary to break apart the various facets of the food system in order to really see their impact in order to work toward change. Therein lies one of the biggest obstacles in fixing our food system. In order to truly fix the food system and develop a sustainable model we need to look at the system as a whole due to its complex web of connections. However, in doing so the task becomes so overwhelming and requires the cooperation of so many individuals it makes it seemingly impossible. Therefore, we need to break down the food system into its parts and individually evaluate those environmental effects. We can then focus on small victories across the food system and produce ripple effects with positive reactions.

A RICH BREEDING GROUND

Animal husbandry is one area that has a huge environmental impact. Our country is not a culture of vegetarians. As Mark Bittman recently pointed out in his new series in the *New York Times*, "Americans eat about the same amount of meat as we have for some time, about eight ounces a day, roughly twice the global average. At about 5 percent of the world's population, we 'process' (that is, grow and kill) nearly 10 billion animals a year, more than 15 percent of the world's total."[30] This issue is growing on a global level. For developing countries, the consumption of meat is considered a sign of affluence. According to the World Watch Institute, around half the meat produced for consumption happens on a factory farm. The Food and Water Watch states that in the last decade the number of livestock on factory farms has increased by 20%, the size of pork farms has doubled to average around 10,000 head; poultry has followed suit with farms cresting on average at 750,000 birds.[31] This facet of the food industry epitomizes the need for understanding the relationship between sound environmental practices and corresponding farming methods. The land can only sustain so much. Think about it like a Bounty Quicker-Picker-Upper commercial. We can keep improving the strength of the towel with all of our technology; but, it still can only withstand so much and,

81

eventually, even the Bounty towel will break. The beef and pork industries, the poultry industry, and the fishing industry play an ever-increasing role in providing the food that feeds the world; their practices, from start to finish, have possibly the most significant impact on the environment.

Frankly, none of these industries function in a way that is good for the environment. Like the vegetable/commodity crop farms, these "manufacturers" are capable of changing their methods and switching to earth-friendly farming. Granted, this change would seriously alter how food gets to the market; but, keep in mind, this is how they started—with thousands of years of earth-friendly farming. As the drive for faster, better, cheaper developed in our general industries, we lumped food in with them. Yes, I do realize there were social changes that coincided with this industrialization of the food industry, such as single-parent households and dual-working households. I also realize that the industry was providing what the public desired; which, of course, is an excellent example of the power of consumer demand to change how an industry operates.

THE CHAIN REACTION

In altering the supply to meet the demand, we changed how we thought about food and eating. How do we get it back? It will take another change of mind-set, a lot of work, and probably the assistance of government subsidies for that or any transition to happen successfully. This change is not just a romantic ideal though; it is a necessity and an attainable goal with the right kind of approach.

Eric Schlosser (*Fast Food Nation*) and Michael Pollan (*The Omnivore's Dilemma*, *In Defense of Food*) break down the

82

beef industry and its effects on the environment in their bestselling books. It is clear that the industry most severely affected, perhaps even devastated, if the country's farmers—primarily those dealing in livestock—began farming green would be the fast-food industry. I recall a recent conversation with one of my chef friends. We were discussing the pros and cons of grass-fed, local beef and my ability to put my beliefs into practice because I run a chef-owned restaurant. We also discussed the quality differences between the two and the possibility of reintegrating a grass-fed product into the market on a large scale based on taste alone. The taste discussion has a simple answer, a great product prepared by good cooks can shoulder a successful integration and eventually increase demand followed by an increase in supply. The cost factor is the one that hinders the debate, for the moment.

By running a chef-owned restaurant I am not accountable to a corporate bean-counter or shareholders. I can justify a higher food cost because of the type of restaurant I have. I should qualify this by explaining my food cost varied only one point in five years, which was right in line with industry average. This remained true even after eliminating industrial and processed products and concentrating on buying as much local product as possible. Now, as this project is reaching the two-year mark, I am proud to report my food cost is on the decline. We are down 4.5 percentage points, after being open seven years (which is like 120 in restaurant years), and my staff has become more proficient in our nose-to-tail usage of product. Through this total usage we are able to decrease our per pound cost on the front end, by purchasing a less-handled product. While we are experiencing some increase in prices due to changes in some basic commodities such as recycled aluminum foil, organic flour and sugar, organic beans, etc., we have still managed to reduce costs. The steady increase in worldwide food prices over the last few years and the bleak projections for future prices mean any savings is invaluable. A recent post from the *Los Angeles Times* gives a shortened overview of the myriad reports regarding worldwide increased food prices.

> Food costs will rise as much as 4% this year, more than the 2% to 3% estimated last month, after a surge in prices for farm goods, the U.S. Department of Agriculture said Thursday. Forecasts were raised for meat, eggs, cooking oils, fruits and vegetables, sweets and cereals and baked goods as food inflation accelerated at the fastest pace since reaching a 28-year high in 2008, the USDA said in a report. Higher costs for corn, the primary feed for pigs and chickens, may boost pork prices as much as 6.5% and eggs 4.5%.[32]

The Food and Agriculture Organization of the United Nations reports on the cost of food worldwide:

> By mid-2008, international food prices had skyrocketed to their highest level in 30 years. This, coupled with the global economic downturn, pushed millions more people into poverty and hunger.

> In December 2010, the FAO food price index had risen above its 2008 peak, and

in January 2011, it had increased by 3.4 percent.[33]

Many reports are pointing toward this increase of food prices as a contributing cause for the recent uprisings in the Middle East.

This report shares an interesting and contradictory point: Even with rising food prices, commercial meat for the restaurant industry is unbelievably inexpensive right now. Why is that?

Our Fast-Food Nation

Consumers have gravitated toward cheap, quick meals because they needed (or, maybe more accurately, wanted) the convenience. As we increased our two-job households and moms continued to enter the workforce, the fast-food industry was there to answer the call. As the percentage of income spent on food decreased, we wanted cheaper options and the fast-food industry provided them. As Eric Schlosser says in *Fast Food Nation*:

> In 1970, Americans spent about $6 billion on fast food; in 2000, they spent more than $110 billion. Americans now spend more money on fast food than on higher education, personal computers, computer software, or new cars. They spend more on fast food than on movies, books, magazines, newspapers, videos, and recorded music—combined.[34]

In 2010 Americans spent almost $170 billion on fast food. Even while mired in the worst recession/depression since before the fast-food industry emerged, sales have been sustained. In fact, the industry has shown growth at a faster rate than before the recession struck. According to the RNCOS Industry Research Solutions 2010 market report, this growth was greater than 4%. One particularly shocking statistic was that the sale of hamburgers alone in the United States was around $75 billion. **SEVENTY-FIVE BILLION DOLLARS IN HAMBURGERS** in one year.[35] The more ground beef the fast-food industry uses, the lower the cost will be for other cuts from the cow. The demand for ground beef is high, which means the supply of the "high end" cuts has increased as well. Therefore, the cost of those prized cuts that are now potentially considered "leftovers" goes down. Are they really "leftover cuts"? No, but when you consider that the drive for industrialization was in large part due to the demand from key buyers (i.e., fast food), and those buyers want ground beef, then two tenderloins, two strips, and two rib eyes become leftovers. I mention only these because they are the main cuts used in restaurants.

Government subsidies of corn and soy make feeding cattle significantly cheaper, which, in turn, means the cows are fattened up more quickly, cost less to bring to slaughter, and are sold more cheaply. This cost-cutting is passed on to enable the fast-food industry to keep their prices low. Although you could also argue that it could have been the demand of the fast-food industry for cheap product that forced the integration of the cheap supply. The cost of fossil fuels also plays a major role in keeping food cheap, as was evident by the recent increase in all commodity crops, some processed food, and general food prices across the board when gas prices skyrocketed in 2008. Do you know which prices stayed exactly the same, during that time? Local food.

BEEF

While this "cost-effectiveness" might sound appealing, we have to consider the hidden costs—the impact of this cheap production. The meat industry is indirectly accountable for many environmental detriments. To me, the most frightening impact of the beef industry is that it is responsible for 18% of the greenhouse gas emissions in our country.[36] That is more than the transportation industry! It is the second highest contributor of atmosphere-altering methane gas, which is twenty times as damaging as carbon dioxide.[37] The majority of this gas is released via animal emissions. Yes, I mean cow farts, burps, and waste. Bovine belches actually contain the higher concentration of methane. That study doesn't even bring into account the amount of grain used for feed and the resulting nitrous oxide released into the environment from industrial agriculture, a gas that is 300 times more potent than carbon dioxide for global warming.[38] Earlier in this chapter I mentioned the need to look beyond the climate change discussion. It still must be part of the discussion, just not the only part.

I once had a good discussion with a new cattle farmer just developing a herd south of Nashville. He was trying to sell me his beef, which is grown on an organic, sustainable farm. They limit the size of their herd, rotate their feeding grounds, and grow all their own food. They understand what chefs need and are working with their processor to get the cuts just the way their customers want them. They are using the entire cow, from nose to tail, and have found secondary uses for the excess product. I was thoroughly impressed. I asked what kind of grass he was growing for feed and his pasture rotation, hay supplements, etc., and his response was his cattle were fed corn. A little taken aback after his big sustainable pitch, I asked how he felt about the amount of gases produced by his cattle eating corn. He scoffed at the greenhouse gas comment and gave a quick rebuttal of how every human puts out CO_2 when we breathe. He explained that the cows love the corn they are fed, and if you let them eat on their own they will gravitate toward corn. We left our conversation there, but his corn comment/argument got me wondering. Was the introduction of corn to cows something that happened by accident? It's quite possible a cow kept getting loose and the farmer noticed it kept moseying on over to the corn fields. When the cow was finally processed they noticed that the cow had great marbling (fat content) and could be cut with a butter knife. In actuality, the process of feeding corn to cows was started by the original farmers in the Corn Belt to use up their excess corn.[39]

The really good news is this local farmer is actually one of three or four new cattle farmers in our area who are growing in a sustainable manner—either organically or, even better, organically and grass finished. We have to recognize the small victories right now. Is the corn-fed aspect of his operation a deterrent for chefs looking to source environmentally sound product? Maybe, but in some areas organic, local corn-fed beef might be the only product available. It's still a better choice than industrial sources. Also, the grass-finished beef might not always be a quality product (see chapter 3, "Local and Sustainable," for more on this topic).

The Financial Costs

The significance of this story is that the farmers are seeing the demand for healthy, environmentally friendly beef and are changing their operations to meet the demand. That yields one very important result: the supply will go up and the cost will go down. My beef cost had been incredibly high—probably twice the going rate for conventional restaurant steaks. Every time I sold a steak I lost money. (Since I began working on this book, my beef cost has come down such that it is almost equivalent to the cost of USDA prime industrial steaks.) Technically, I don't charge what I should; but, that is by choice, and I am able to cover the difference in other ways. Besides, we are already considered—although I am at a loss for why—very pricey. It is not unusual for restaurants to have a dish on their menu for which they can't recover the cost, though not typically with such a significant shortfall. However, I am providing the public with a high-quality, grass-finished beef that has more flavor and is a better product than industrial beef. It is environmentally friendly and it is a local steak. To me, that makes it all worth the expense.

Using a proper menu mix balancing high-cost items with low-cost items allows you to stay within your food budget and absorb the extra expense. But we shouldn't allow cost to be the determining factor. Quality and flavor should be our priority. I will put my steak up against an industrially grown steak and win nine times out of ten. The marbling of these cattle is superb; and, for the most part, that has been the biggest difference between the corn/grain-fed and grass-finished varieties. We have grown accustomed to beef that can be cut with a butter knife. And why not? It is true that it is amazingly tender; but, it's also true that this meat offers little flavor and usually tastes like corn or just the seasoning and whatever was used to cook it, which is typically butter. And, although everybody knows that butter makes everything better, do you really want to have to cook your steak in it to make that steak flavorful?

The Environmental Costs

We are just scratching the surface discussing the number of environmental concerns surrounding the industrial cattle system. So far we have focused on the climate change issues related to greenhouse gases from livestock production. There are many more direct and indirect effects, some very similar to the issues with commodity vegetable crops. Deforestation, for one, is just as prevalent in cattle farming as it is in commodity farming—the larger the herd, the more space needed. To get more space, burn down some forest. An excerpt from Richard Robbins, found on the GlobalIssues.org website, states:

> Cattle raising has also been criticized for its role in the destruction of tropical forests. Hundreds of thousands of acres of tropical forests in Brazil, Guatemala, Costa Rica, and Honduras, to name just a few countries, have been leveled to create pasture for cattle. Since most of the forest is cleared by burning, the extension of cattle pasture also creates carbon dioxide, and, according to some environmentalists, contributes significantly to global warming.[40]

Erosion is another factor livestock production and vegetable farming hold in common. In commodity vegetable farming the constant use of fertilizers and pesticides kills the humus in the soil, decreasing the strength of the soil. This decrease in strength means the soil cannot absorb water and stay moist and is subsequently easily washed away. On industrial animal farms, the waste from the animals is mixed with water and sprayed onto the surrounding land. The concentrated waste changes from a beneficial fertilizer to a harmful humus killer in these mass concentrations. The soil result is the same. "Currently, the average rate of soil erosion on U.S. cropland is seven tons per acre per year."[41] Thankfully, recent regulations are requiring improved waste management, some of which prevent manure spraying as a waste-removal technique altogether. These regulations are for new construction.

One of the major environmental concerns comes from the Confined Animal Feedlot Operations (CAFOs) used to fatten the cattle before slaughter—the places that produce the aforementioned concentrated waste. In order to pack these animals together and prevent the spread of illness and disease, they are given antibiotics. Currently, 70–80% of the antibiotics being produced in this country go to animal husbandry.[42] The trickle-down effect from these antibiotics is being seen in medical facilities around the country. As the cattle build a tolerance to these drugs, so do we. Then the bugs become more resilient. Again we thank Brillat-Savarin for his "we are what we eat" observation. Infectious diseases are no longer being controlled with the same antibiotics. As we eat these antibiotics on a regular basis we slowly build up resistance to their effects. Yet that is not the only way these unintentional antibiotics get into our system. As the water table near these farms becomes polluted, the waste ends up in the ocean, is eaten by microbes, and travels up the food chain back to us. The viruses that make us sick have already survived these antibiotics; so, as we administer more to cure ourselves, the strains of viruses are able to resist them. Basically, we stay sicker with a more powerful bug.

Many more environmental concerns arise as cattle reach the CAFOs. Pollution in several forms is an increasing problem generated by these facilities, with erosion being one by-product. It is estimated that CAFOs produce as much waste as a small city. The waste is collected in pools throughout the feedlots after it is removed from the pens. "Giant commercial confined livestock and poultry operations produce half a billion tons of manure each year, more than three times as much as that produced by the entire U.S. population."[43] The cattle wade through their own feces while feeding in their cramped environment. The CAFOs claim there are treatments in place to make this waste safe for disposal, and new regulations are forcing a more environmentally safe solution, but for the most part it ends up finding its way into our groundwater, causing contamination and carrying chemicals into the water stream. Dried particles also make it into the air, decreasing the value of the surrounding land and sickening residents.[44] CAFOs take up land, killing any biodiversity that may have been in that area and destroying the land for future generations. "Livestock's presence in vast tracts of land and its demand for feed crops also contribute to biodiversity loss; 15 out of 24 important ecosystem services are assessed as in decline, with livestock identified as a culprit."[45]

Some issues I've covered more in depth than others and, again, I haven't even scratched the surface of the concerns surrounding industrial beef production. The information is easily accessible. From a chef's perspective the only benefit to a CAFO is the ability to get a case of tenderloins the next day with a quick phone call. The negatives far outweigh the positives in this scenario. When you look into how that case of tenderloins got to you, how can you justify putting that on the plate?

The Solution

There is of course an answer to industrial beef production. Buy local or grass-finished beef. When we say grass-finished we mean an animal that has been raised on grass for its whole life until it is processed. The highlights of the environmental benefits of grass-finished beef are: a significant decrease in greenhouse gas emissions from lack of travel, lack of fossil fuel use in production, lack of unnatural animal emissions from a proper diet, lack of emissions from the feed production, proper waste disposal, decreased erosion, and reduction of water supply contamination. The health benefits from grass-finished beef include: fewer food safety issues from cattle raised in a healthier environment, minimal-to-no use of hormones for growth or antibiotics to prevent disease, a product that is healthier for your body due to an increase in beneficial fats, and decreased food safety issues from processing at a small or mid-sized plant that is not run like an assembly line.[46] We could also get into the benefits for the local economy, the health of the workers, the value of the land, and more.

So that answer, again, is to buy grass-fed, start-to-finish, local beef. A task that, currently, is much easier said than done. As we've discussed previously, the most important part of sourcing your food is to ensure the best quality. That is your primary job as a chef. Now, as a chef, your secondary job is to make food costs fit your budget, making money for the business. When you make the transition to buying locally you will encounter the cost dilemma we've already discussed. But there is another initial downside to buying local meat. In order to permanently make the change, it becomes necessary to be more flexible in your offerings. Again, the ability to call and get twelve tenderloins the next day is gone. Now that we at *tāyst* have immersed ourselves in our quest for local markets, versatility and flexibility are a requirement for being successful. Our answer to this problem is using the menu to our advantage, really selling people on the importance of these items as local steak or local pork. I am very proud to say that I finally have managed to ensure that all land-based meat featured on our menu is grown in our region.

CHICKEN

Chicken was the last item, at that time, preventing me from entirely becoming a protein locavore (besides duck and foie gras). You can have a menu without duck and foie; but, generally speaking, you can't have one without chicken. Two different poultry farmers were launching their farms a few years ago and I had the opportunity to sample their birds. Both were delicious. The big problem we initially faced with chicken was that we could only get chicken that was affordable (the key word here) sporadically. Let's quickly define "affordable." We discussed cost related to beef already; but, chicken is a different bag because chicken is seen as a "high-profit/low-cost" dish—low-cost for the restaurant and the consumer, but still very profitable. At first we were looking at $4 to $5 per pound on chickens, quite an increase from the occasional high price of $1

94

per pound for industrial chicken. We would receive twenty here or thirty there, and then that would be it for a couple of months. We had one farm that started out with good product at a good price and quickly realized the market potential. They overpromised, started buying birds raised differently from neighbors, their quality diminished, and then that farm disappeared. It popped back up a year or so later in the CSA market. I had long discussions with the potential new local providers in preparation for the upcoming season. At that time we were using about thirty chickens a week. We agreed to take about that many every other week, alternating between them, with the understanding that this number could go up or down. On the weeks that my orders were down they would hold those chickens back, which created a surplus that allowed me to get chickens through the winter as well.

Is Free-Range Really Free?

The reason I can't get them to raise chickens in the winter is because all these beautiful local birds are pasture chickens. Basically, that means each day they are released from a mobile, double-wide hen house (or something like it) to graze on fresh pasture. They spend the day outside, living the way they were meant to live, and eating what they were meant to eat and then head on back into their mobile houses. They also tend to grow exceptionally slowly in the cold weather months increasing the cost factor. It is the opposite of what industrial chickens, including those listed as free-range are given. Just in case you are not aware . . . industrial free-range chickens with the pretty farm pasture picture on the packaging are not allowed outside until they are six weeks old, then a door is opened to an outside pen with about ten square feet of space. Unfortunately, by the time the chickens can go outside they are accustomed to staying inside and do not use the door. According to the USDA, a bird or egg can be labeled free-range if it has "access to the outside."[47] The same follows suit for the egg industry. The hen houses do not vary much from the poultry houses in theory. Obviously they do have a different living system on the inside for egg laying and removal. Our egg sourcing follows the same storyline we've seen for chicken and beef. We started out with trickles and then built up support solely to rely on pasture-raised hens providing wondrous eggs that vary with the seasons.

Working example time: The egg guy I'd been using for a couple of years quit coming to town, and his farm was too far to go and pick up the eggs. I had to scramble (pun intended) to find eggs any way I could. I was getting a couple dozen here, maybe five dozen there. Finally, after I had sufficiently got the word out about my egg dilemma in the farmer circles I was put in touch with a farmer who was selling eggs at the local markets. I had no previous dealings with him and gave him my usual rundown of questions. He had all the right answers and we started to do business. What happened next? Massive nationwide egg recall; you might remember it. All of a sudden everybody wanted local eggs. I called up to place an order. It is important to give the farmers a little heads up when you want to buy 20–30 dozen eggs. Not only will they keep them aside for you, they won't be caught off guard at the market and will still have enough for their customers. His initial reaction to my order was negative. He said he couldn't fill the order. Then he quickly backtracked and said no worries. Well, I go to pick up my eggs and get back to the shop. A case of industrial, perfectly sized, all-white eggs. As in all business there are those who will try to get one over on you, who are less scrupulous. The lesson: know your farmer. Also, even after all these years and a powerful infrastructure it is important to be flexible and have multiple avenues for all of your products.

PORK

I think the quickest way to start the local menu transition is by finding local farms for pork. The push for heritage breeds has really taken hold throughout the country. In all the markets I've visited, pork has always been the most prevalent meat available. Seriously though, should we have expected anything else? As Homer Simpson says, pork is "the glorious mythical beast that gives us chops and bacon," or something like that. It is also great to see that raising pork in an environmentally responsible manner has helped to bring back breeds that were almost extinct—breeds like Tamworth, Red Wattle, and Berkshire that were prevalent before World War II. Let's not leave out the European variety the furry and fatty, Mangalitsa.

Along with the other meat industries, varieties of pork have been bred out and replaced with an industrial version, which is a gigantic, lean beast that will stay moist no matter how much you cook it. It has been bred to get fat quick and stay tender. The irony of using the terms "get fat quick" is that the industrial breed has a very low fat content. The fat content has also been decreased during this genetic streamlining—an unfortunate trait due to the fact that fat is flavor. The quality of industrial chickens has actually followed the same path. They have been bred to be a "gigantic chicken McNugget" as Robert Kenner, director of the film, "Food Inc.," said in an interview on PBS. He goes on to say these chickens become so fat (meaning big) so fast they no longer have the ability to stand.

In both cases the animals are raised in CAFOs. The difference between the pork and chicken CAFOs compared to the beef CAFOs is that the animals never see the light of day. At least cattle start out in pastures. One of the other really nasty results of industrialized pork production is the smell produced from the houses and the waste pools on these farms. Waste in old pools is still dispersed via spray method. Like cattle CAFOs, regulations have changed to require new construction to incorporate a closed, "environmentally friendly" system. The jury is still out on that claim. In all cases, a stench emanates from the buildings where the pigs are confined. The buildings are fitted with air circulation vents in order to keep the gases from collecting. They are also backed up with alarms and generators not only to keep track of gas levels, but to prevent any power outage that would result in a loss of pigs. Pig farmers know the gases emitted from pig waste can be toxic if not ventilated, yet they confine these animals anyway. We know this is bad, they know it is bad by their attempts to control it, yet we still support this type of farm. It is equally astonishing to me that it has been shown that keeping pigs outside in a rotating system will not only eliminate these smells, it will retain, and even increase, profits in an environmentally sound manner—better for the animals, better for the farmer, better for the community.

Look, I'm not shocking the world with the information we've been discussing. To me, it's pretty obvious that industrial meat production is not environmentally friendly. I think in this day and age most people are aware at some level of the detriment to using this style of production. Also, I feel that there are still many folks, in the business and out, who know but don't quite realize the vast scope of effect of industrial animal husbandry. As with all the information in this book, I hope to connect the dots and spark the desire in you to find out the finer details. Use the resources in the appendix, be the expert in your kitchen and at the table.

Chapter Five
Water-Based Proteins

To this point we have concentrated on land animals and the impact the industrial raising of cattle has on the surrounding environment. It is important to also address the other animal-based protein—fish—and the effects non-sustainable practices have on our waterways. A recent article in *OnEarth*, an online magazine, states that "fishing feeds three billion people. It provides half the animal protein in the diets of 400 million of the world's poorest citizens, and the livelihoods of 500 million people depend on the trade."[48] This doesn't even account for the meat eaters in developed countries who occasionally eat fish. As we mentioned in the previous chapter, there is a shift occurring in developing countries to a more meat-based diet; but, for the majority of the world's 7 billion people, fish is a major part of their diet. Perhaps this is one of the reasons that what is going on beneath the ocean's surface might be the scariest environmental issue of all.

Again the discussion of environmentally sound eating forces us to look globally. I think this could be one of the hardest concepts to grasp. I continually talk about the need to source locally and eat locally and about the benefits that will come from making a greener society; yet it is vital for us to be concerned on a global scale as well. "Presently about 40% of the world's population lives within 100 kilometers of the coast."[49] That means that 60% of the population would have to eliminate ocean fish from their diets in order to enable a local, sustainable food system. That is never going to happen. People love fish in all shapes, sizes, and preparations. The fish discussion brings up the issue of what I call "traveling sustainability." We will discuss this more in the chapter on defining sustainability, but it is basically the use of sustainable product that is from far away. In a global economy the discussion of a sustainable food system will have to incorporate food from far away at some point. And, as we previously stated, the trade of products between foodsheds, or regions, is part of the cause for economic globalization. So this is one of the examples where local sources are typically sustainable, but not all sustainable sources are local.

We are part of an ecosystem, we do not live in a vacuum and what we do locally does have a global impact. It is my firm belief that we can fix our country and the world, one by one, a time. It will take just one community to become a model and show success in its ability to be self-sustaining. The reality is the world as a whole is one large community made up of smaller ones. The ocean is a great example of this relationship. It is broken into many small ecosystems (communities) that are self-sufficient and sustainable—wetlands, coral reefs, deep water, etc.—but they are also affected by what is happening across the ocean in another community. The disruption of the wetlands will eventually have a negative impact on the coral reefs, which will, in turn, affect the deepest parts of the sea. We are watching this happen every day in our oceans.

According to the American Association of the Advancement of Science, the world fish populations are one-sixth of what they were one hundred years ago. In the seafood documentary "The End of the Line," scientists predict that if we continue fishing as we are now, we will see the end of most seafood by 2048.[50] A sentiment reiterated by many, including ocean advocate Sylvia Earle. I would say that is clear evidence we are fishing in an unsustainable manner. How have we gone from endless bounty to a depleted supply that is not sufficiently regenerating itself? As I sat back to think about this, I realized that I haven't caught a fish while surfcasting on Nantucket in a long time, a realization similar to the one had by *The End of the Line* author Charles Clover, which sparked his journey. We used to go out in the summer when I was a kid and we almost always caught some fish. It was easy to tell when they were biting—through slicks formed from their feeding, birds diving, or literally seeing them in the ocean. I vividly remember surfing one late afternoon and paddling back out as a wave came toward me. In the wave I saw a large school of bluefish. I caught the next wave in, ran home, grabbed my pole, and soon had dinner for the evening. I go back to Nantucket every year and I am even fortunate enough lately to be able to spend a good amount of time there in the summers. I haven't caught a fish from the beach (not for lack of trying), nor have I seen the signs in probably the last fifteen years that the fish are biting. We are talking bluefish, too, a species that hasn't been significantly affected by overfishing . . . yet. We have a very serious problem.

Not everyone is on the same page regarding the pending devastation of the fishing industry. In a *New York Times* opinion piece, Ray Hilborn stated that the catch numbers causing the concern for overfishing are exaggerated and a correlation between catch and amount of fish is impossible to gauge since the onset of fisheries management. In fact, most fish populations have begun to stabilize and in the United States they are actually replenishing.[51] He does admit that certain species are suffering serious shortages, but argues that losing a few species is a necessary and acceptable sacrifice if it means more sustainable practices in the long run and the betterment of humans and the environment.

However, the majority of marine scientists believe we are in dire straits. We have reached the point that 70% of the world's fish stocks are depleted. "Unsustainable fishing caused by poor fisheries management and wasteful destructive fishing practices is decimating the world fisheries, marine habitats, and killing billions of unwanted fish and other marine animals."[52] When pollutants and contaminants from industrial runoff are killing whole communities (i.e., the dead zone in the Gulf of Mexico), our ocean life stands little chance for survival.

FISHING FROM THE WRONG SIDE OF THE BOAT

According to the World Wildlife Fund (WWF) the major pitfalls of the fishing industry are related to technology, perverse subsidies, partnerships, pirate fishing, bycatch, destructive practices, and poor fishery management.[53] Much like with industrial farming, the information surrounding these issues has increased tenfold since I began this project. For starters, the book and documentary *The End of the Line* do a great job covering precisely these issues through an exposé on the tuna industry. Other sources such as the online program from the Blue Ocean Institute and the Chef's Collaborative website titled "Green Chefs, Blue Ocean" provide an educational class focusing on the issues as well as solutions to the seafood dilemma. I will summarize what each of these aforementioned terms means and what they are doing to the world's fish supply. The description of these terms is a compilation from the Blue Ocean Institute, the Marine

Stewardship Council, the World Wildlife Fund, the Monterey Bay Aquarium, and the Food and Water Watch.

Technology

Technological advancement is arguably the greatest achievement of the human race, but has brought with it countless unforeseen adverse effects. I think everyone will agree in the case of genetically modified food, fertilizers, and pesticides, we leapt before we looked. Through technological advances we have been able to develop bigger nets to put on faster boats. The makeup of the nets themselves has been altered dramatically with a stronger plastic variety—one that is nearly invisible and eliminates the problems of nylon netting. Boats have added bigger motors and onboard refrigeration units allowing them to fish longer and farther from land. The uses of radar, sonar, satellites, and airplanes have taken the guesswork out of fishing. The number and size of fleets has increased considerably in the last 30–40 years.

Subsidies and Partnerships

Much in the same way as in agriculture we are using taxpayer dollars to subsidize the fishing fleets. This subsidization is keeping fleets much larger than necessary out in the water. As it stands now, the global fishing fleet is two and a half times larger than what the oceans can support. Combine this with unfair partnerships in which wealthy countries pay lump sums to the governments of poorer countries in order to fish in their waters. "Under these deals, the recipient government is paid a lump sum to allow foreign boats to fish in their waters."[54] Widely criticized as a contributing factor to overfishing, a threat to the food security of developing countries, and an obstacle to the development of local fishing industries, these deals are ineffectively regulated and hardly controlled.[55]

Pirate Fishing

Pirate fishing—illegal, unreported, and unregulated (IUU) fishing—is happening all over the world. It is estimated that 30% of all fish sent to market is caught illegally, although it would be almost impossible to get a completely accurate figure since pirate fishing (obviously) goes unreported.[56] This also encompasses the practice of name variation. The best example is the Patagonian Toothfish, a species close to extinction that for years was listed on menus as Chilean Sea Bass. Let me clarify that these are not two species, but one with a second name used for marketing purposes only. Even now, with the widely known fact that it is illegal to catch and serve this fish, I see it on menus.

Bycatch

Bycatch is probably the most destructive result of the modern fishing industry. As we have increased our efficiency in catching the fish that *is* sought we are also increasing the frequency of catching the fish we don't seek, or "bycatch." This bycatch is typically juvenile or injured fish that will die before they are returned to the ocean. According to the WWF, bycatch results in the deaths of 300,000 small whales, dolphins, and porpoises each year. Additionally, 250,000 loggerhead and critically endangered leatherback turtles are caught on longlines, twenty-six species of seabird are now close to extinction, 89% of hammerhead and 80% of thresher sharks have been eliminated, and shrimp trawlers are catching close to 35,000,000 juvenile red snappers each year. And "high grading," or the discarding of lesser quality catch in order to get the highest return for quotas, is potentially the worst in my eyes. [Sidebar: Just recently it has been reported that once-decimated fish populations are now being restored to sustainable levels through properly enforced regulations, one great example that we can turn things around.] We have already reached a point in which 90% of the big fish in the oceans are gone. This is having a devastating effect on the delicate balance of that ecosystem. There are very obvious and completely avoidable reasons for the bycatch. A number of the fishing techniques that are in use at this time have been "over improved." The traditional practices of bottom trawling, gillnets, longlines, purse seines, and dredging, which have been in use for hundreds or even thousands of years, are no longer a safe way to catch fish. By combining these age-old techniques with technological advancements like the ones previously listed, the resulting damages have made these techniques harmful not just to fish populations but the environment in which they live. Dredges and trawls have gotten larger and stronger, lines have gotten longer, nets have gotten more efficient. We have become better at catching the fish we want; however, we are also better at catching the fish we don't want.

Destructive Fishing Practices

Dredging. Another cause for the fish disappearance is the use of destructive fishing practices. As I stated earlier, I grew up on Nantucket Island, which—hands down, by far, no competition— has the best bay scallops in the world. Nantucket is a great example of a small community that depleted its environment and as a result seriously damaged its natural resources. The scallop population has been tragically compromised. The chosen form of fishing for scallops is dredging, which has been used for hundreds of years. The by-product of dredging is the destruction of the aquaculture or sea grasses on the sea bed. The loss of these grasses changed the ecosystem of the floor in the harbors and, combined with unregulated fishing, the scallop population significantly declined. In the early nineteen hundreds scallop men were bringing in approximately 150,000 bushels a year in bay scallops. In 1980–81 the take was 117,000 bushels and in 1999 it was only 6,800 bushels.[57] In an effort to stop this depletion, regulations and quotas were instituted. As of the first decade of 2000, quotas were ranging between 5,000 and 15,000 bushels per year, alternating the harbors open for fishing. The Saving SeaFood website tells us that "island scallopers hauled in just over 6,916 bushels of the succulent shellfish between Nov. 1, 2010, and the end of March 2011. That's a far cry from the 18,116 bushels harvested the previous season, but better than early predictions following a dismal recreational scalloping season."[58]

Trawling. A close cousin to dredging is bottom trawling. In the beginning, bottom trawling stayed away from reefs and rocks because the trawls would get caught, torn, or destroyed. Now they are built with heavy wheels on the bottom and reefs are no longer a danger to their nets. The trawls roll right over the reefs, destroying them as they go. Coral reefs do not grow back on their own, as explained by the Coral Reef Alliance: "When coral reefs die, fish populations disappear; beaches and shorelines are damaged. Unprotected by breakwaters, fragile land areas become vulnerable to erosion, saltwater intrusion and destruction from waves. For an already damaged reef, regeneration is very slow taking several decades, even under ideal conditions."[59]

Cyanide fishing. Another quite disturbing technique is called cyanide fishing. The water is squirted with cyanide to stun the fish, making them easy to catch. This practice also provides live reef fish for those restaurants that have the little fish tanks in the front, which means we are experiencing an unintended exposure to cyanide as well. The cyanide technique also destroys a yard of reef for every fish that is caught.

Dynamite. Finally, and probably the most unnecessarily destructive technique, is dynamite. I don't believe that needs any further explanation.

A SEA OF CHANGE

Negative, negative, negative. Almost everything we have covered so far is negative. Unfortunately, sometimes negativity and shock value are what it takes to initiate serious change. Science shows how badly our food system is in need of help. But there is still hope. The positive side of all this doom and gloom is that there are solutions. Fishing practices have only become significantly damaging when combined with our subsidized, technical prowess. This is a trend that can be reversed. We are starting to see change in the techniques available to fisheries in order to minimize or eliminate the environmental damage that comes from industrialization and overfishing. We are also already seeing positive results from some of the implemented regulations.

New and Improved Methods

Scientists are working with fisheries in order to develop, test, and implement new fishing gear—gear such as hook and line trolling in which tow lines are set at different depths—a higher cost technique, yes, but one that is very eco-friendly and ultimately has a lower environmental cost. Hook and line with a rod in which only a few hooks are used is another option. Harpooning, traps and pots, and eco-friendly seining, fishing with special nets, are some of the other techniques. Improvements to the current gear are also being investigated, such as circle hooks, which can be set on tuna longlines at greater depths. The design of the hook prevents the bycatch of turtles and sharks, and knowing that the tuna typically reside below 100 meters decreases the likelihood of trapping unintended sealife. Using these alternatives is showing a 90% reduction in bycatch so far. Turtle Excluder Devices (TED) in shrimp trawling are a maze of metal grids that allow 97% of turtles to escape. Gillnets are being made safer and more visible. Fisheries are also using chemicals with their net fishing that allow animals using echolocation to detect nets, thus avoiding them. The technology that got us into this destructive problem can also be the solution for getting us out if we will start demanding more responsible fishing practices. Ask your seafood purveyor how the fish was caught, it's as important a question as where was it caught.

Fish Farms

There is one more topic in the world of sustainable fishing yet to cover, that of fish farming—a business that was developed in direct response to the issues we are facing in our oceans.

The jury is still out on the impact, although most reports on the early-stage farms are bad and there is no definitive best choice. Have you noticed the underlying theme so far? The color of sustainability in the food system is gray. Later we will discuss in great detail the ambiguities plaguing the efforts for sustainability, but for now it's worth contemplating while you continue reading. The main purpose of fish farming is to supply the world with fish while maintaining the diversity and quantity of species in the ocean. There are basically two types of fish farming: coastal and inland, and they currently supply half of the fish in the market.[60] Within these types there are a number of different styles of farms. Environmentally speaking, the level of impact is dependent on the species being farmed and the intensity of the operation.

Coastal farms usually involve a type of carnivorous fish like salmon, bass, or barramundi kept in pens with coastal nets. As with the CAFOs on land, the fish in these tight quarters require antibiotics in order to prevent disease; just as with the cattle, they are developing resistance to the antibiotics. They are burdened with not quite similar yet equally harmful waste disposal issues and suffer from potential pollution issues as well. Their waste carries diseases and chemicals into the open oceans, polluting not just the surrounding waters, but coastlines across the oceans. *Science Daily* recently reported on a study experimenting with fish farm waste scenarios: "Concentrated waste plumes from fish farms could travel significant distances to reach coastlines."[61] As with all animals in captivity farmed fish are susceptible to disease. Salmon farms are (in)famous for their sea lice, which, due to escaping fish, are now being found on wild catch. These diseases have the capability of wiping out entire populations of fish.[62] A few years ago the Chilean-based farm-raised salmon industry

110

experienced this very issue—a diseased population that decimated its numbers—and the cost of farm-raised fish skyrocketed to a rate that was only pennies from the price of wild salmon.[63] The most important fact in the farm-raising operations is that these are carnivorous fish eating fish meal made from wild fish. It takes five pounds of wild fish meal to raise one pound of salmon.[64] Isn't that completely defeating the purpose? It is simply counter-intuitive to kill perfectly good wild catch and turn it into lesser farm-raised product.

Inland farms are receiving a mixed response. Again, their effectiveness is determined by the species and the intensity of the operation. The two major freshwater farmed fish are catfish and trout. Unfortunately, neither, save a few exceptions (or should I say *exceptional* companies), seems to be farming with the environmental impact in mind. Catfish farms harvest their fish and then, in order to kill any remaining life, pour pesticides into the water that, shockingly, can cause paralysis in humans if inhaled. The fish are packed full of antibiotics and we already know the problems associated with that. The trout industry is troublingly similar to the chicken industry. They are typically raised in concrete pens or streams and the water is circulated, then cleaned. However, chemicals are used in conjunction with antibiotics in order to increase output. Like salmon, trout are carnivorous; they only need three pounds of wild fish to make the meal to raise one pound of trout.[65]

Fish farming is not all bad. There are sustainable farms sprouting up inland and on coastlands—trout farms like Sunburst Trout Farm just outside of Asheville, North Carolina, Australis Aquaculture in Massachusetts, and ocean farms like Kona Blue off the coast of Hawaii—that are learning from the mistakes we have made and turning them into advantages by changing the style of farming. The Kona Kampachi fish farmed at Kona Blue are hatched on land and then raised in deep ocean pens, eliminating the need for hormones and antibiotics and the problems of waste.

> By combining a commitment to state-of-the-art marine hatchery science with a carefully selected, pristine deep ocean grow-out site, Kona Blue can raise Kona Kampachi® without depleting wild fish stocks or harming the ocean environment. No genetic engineering, hormones, or preventative antibiotics are used in the process.[66]

I will say that their feed still uses 30% wild catch. This catch is mostly bycatch, which would typically be wasted, so it is not all bad and is a good use of bycatch, which will probably never be completely eliminated. There are farms similar to Kona Blue being started right now to address the issue of the diminishing stores of tuna, which is one of the most overfished species in the world, in hopes that the tuna population can thrive again. Companies are also experimenting with alternate species like Cobia, which naturally grow faster and are more suited to a farming system.[67] It is important to look for farms that voice their sustainable practices and use organic feed. Research your selections.

Sustainable Watch

Perhaps the most important technique to prevent overfishing is the promotion of sustainable fishing. Look at the work of institutions such as the Marine Stewardship Council, the Blue

Ocean Institute, and the Monterey Bay Aquarium in raising the awareness of the importance of purchasing sustainable fish. These groups are researching which techniques are working and which species are in danger. They are providing easy-to-use lists people can check to learn the sustainability of the fish on menus and in stores. They are providing the information people need in order to make responsible choices and ensure that fish will be here for their grandchildren. There is even an app for your iPhone that will instantly tell you if a fish is sustainable. That's progress!

Again, I want to point out how fast ideas are being implemented and how much power this movement wields, or rather, the power wielded by the dollar amount represented. Companies are popping up that I call "fish direct," in which you are basically buying direct from the fisherman via a connector. The connector is a middleman; but, unlike the typical system—where they buy the fish at auction, send it to their warehouse, then a salesman sells the fish, it's fabricated, or cut into portions, and then it's delivered—the fish are shipped via FedEx right from the docks. Ahh, the wonders of the Internet. The fishermen participating in these programs are the ones using the sustainable methods we've covered. That provides us with two benefits, the protection of our fish and the protection of our fishermen. Programs are also being initiated in which there is guaranteed transparency to know how, where, and by whom your fish were caught. Without accurate traceability, provided by websites such as fish2fork.com and the Marine Stewardship Council (MSC)'s new traceability certification, it is nearly impossible for the majority of consumers really know that their fish was properly caught.[68]

Fish Ranching

The most exciting news to recently emerge regarding fish farming is twofold. A new technique called fish ranching has been conceived in which fish, using Pavlov's theory, can be trained to come to a sound played while they are eating. After a few weeks (it varies based on the species), these fish are released into the wild to be the fish they are meant to be. Occasionally, the bell rings and they return to the spot in which they are fed to reinforce the training. When it is time to harvest, the bell is rung, the fish come, a gate is closed, and we have a lot of product with very little environmental impact.[69] The other advancement is that of a vertically integrated multitrophic farm in which a fish farm is on the surface, over a shellfish farm that filters the water, over a grass bed, with crabs and bottom feeders at the end. Essentially this is a biomimicry-inspired fish farm. Biomimicry is the business of mimicking systems of nature for business, using the natural system of life circles in the ocean for a farm blueprint.

Simultaneously, reports have surfaced regarding the state of our oceans from fishing management industries, a few scientists, and U.S. Commerce Secretary Gary Locke. These reports indicate which catches are being increased in some industries around the country. Particularly interesting is that the New England ground fish industry was allowed a 12.5% increase in their catch shares beginning May 1, 2011. This is especially exciting because this particular industry hosts the most horrible unsustainable fish story of all, that of the New England cod—a population so depleted many think it will never recover. Catches are being increased because these reports are showing that the regulations and fishing practices being implemented are, in fact, working. This is a very good sign, one I hope stays true and can be a great example to the rest of the food system.

. As I began to discover all this information about these industries, I was horrified. It didn't matter whether it was beef, fish, corn, or sugar, the facts were pretty clear and the message was the same. Across the board we have to step back and reevaluate how we grow and process our food. The connection between how we treat the earth and its ability to grow our food is inarguable, and we are getting a harsh wake-up call. The world, as a whole, is experiencing growing populations with limited resources and decreasing ability to provide life necessities with those resources. Being "green," "environmentally friendly," or however you want to say it, is directly responsible for the supply and quality of food you have available. That should matter to you. That should affect what you choose to use in your restaurants, cafes, delis, hotels, etc., as well as what you choose to eat out or serve at home. Your purchases will definitely affect how available the right food will be.

Chapter Six
Industrialization

I am sure there are arguments that can be raised for the benefit of industrial farming. In fact, they happen every day on Capitol Hill and are usually quite successful. Proponents of industrial agriculture will make these arguments: Industrial agriculture benefits America by providing increased yields at a faster pace, decreased costs, an economically sustainable food system, increased food safety, increased value in tradable commodities, and greater variety through science. Let's translate these "benefits" into layman's terms. Basically, industrial agriculture provides us with cheap food, removes jobs, boosts the profitability of corporate agricultural and seed companies, and genetically alters our food to fit their system.

I don't believe any of these supposed benefits even comes close to effectively supporting their case. Around the middle of the last century Americans used about one-fifth (or 20%) of their budget on food. By the end of the century that percentage was just shy of 10%.[70] It is true that industrial farming helped the American people by reducing their food expenses, allowing them to use those dollars in other places. Unfortunately, those cuts didn't go to places that actually benefited the families. The decrease in food expenditures was partly a result of subsidies from taxes that provide protection to industrial farmers, which means the money saved on a grocery bill was made up by an increase, maybe not directly, in tax dollars to cover the subsidies. Also, the costs of health care have increased from 5% to 16% per household.[71] Amazingly, the health care expense increase has coincided with the decline of the food cost percentage. Did you know diet-related

116

diseases account for the greatest percentage of medical expenses in our country?

Even though we have seen a saturation of media coverage on this issue, I don't think the message is really getting through that two-thirds of American adults are overweight or obese and the obesity rates in children and teens have doubled in the past few years.[72] Of the Caucasian children born in the year 2000, one-third will have Type-2 diabetes by the time they reach adulthood, and that ratio climbs to one in two for African-Americans and Hispanics.[73] Diet-related diseases also account for as many as 580,000 deaths each year in the United States, beating tobacco, which is responsible for claiming up to 470,000 lives each year. That is thirteen times more deaths than guns and twenty times more than drug use.[74] The makeup of the "Western" or "American" diet contributes to four of the six leading causes of death as well as increasing the risk of other diseases— heart disease, diabetes, obesity, stroke, hypertension, osteoporosis, and many forms of cancer. The cost of treating these diseases is about $617 *billion* annually; although some reports indicate it is closer to $1 trillion annually.[75] According to the USDA, healthier diets could save $71 billion annually by reducing or eliminating medical expenses, lost productivity, and lost lives. That does not even take into consideration the extended costs related to these diseases. Obesity costs alone are estimated at around $117 billion per year.

To put this into perspective, consider this: Our country is home to almost 315 million people, of which, 220 million, give or take, suffer from diet-related diseases that cost our country almost $1 trillion. (Interestingly, the only organization offering numbers on the health care costs associated with our diet that don't correspond with the widely reported data is the USDA, who also happens to regulate how we grow our food and what is okay to eat.) Our country is now almost $14 trillion in debt. It seems to me that we could significantly reduce our health care–related debt simply by changing the way we eat. It seems as if this potential change in health care costs won't have as much of an impact, but you have to remember that healthier people are more productive. There are many benefits to a healthier society.

We should take a cue from the efforts used in the fight against tobacco—learn which strategies were successful and apply those methods to the fight against industrialized food—we have a legitimate chance at winning. The situations are eerily similar. Both industries are tied to the livelihoods of a large number of farmers and are controlled by a few corporations with really good connections and lots of money. A little side note here: One of the real success stories for ex-tobacco farmers has been their recognition of the potential new markets and subsequent transition to organic farming. The anti-tobacco movement focused their education on children, using their influence to bring home the message. Literally, the children brought home the message. The goal in targeting children was twofold: If they could inform children of the health hazards associated with smoking, it would deter them from becoming smokers; in turn, the children would share the message with parents and other family members to convince them to quit smoking.

The CDC reports that governments spend 1,000 times more money to treat diseases than to prevent them—$1,390 per person compared to $1.21 per person.[76] Imagine what we could do with the money saved if we weren't spending so much on curing ailments that could have been prevented! It took us only two generations to get where we are. I believe we

118

can turn it around in our children's lifetimes. It is an overwhelming problem; there is no doubt about that. We can't just stop spending on health care and switch those funds to healthy food subsidies—especially while we are spiraling deeper and deeper into debt. But we can't afford not to find a way to redirect some of our spending to more sensible and responsible uses. So we find another societal issue—debt—directly related to the food system.

CHANGING THE WAY PEOPLE EAT

There is one area in the fight for healthy eating with which I totally disagree. Menu labeling, in my opinion, is and always will be the biggest waste of money spent toward fighting obesity. Caloric information has been available at places like Subway and other fast-food chains for years, and it has changed nothing. In fact, the fast-food industry is actually increasing in business and profits. I remember a marketing lecture from my school days that indicated the practice of listing calories at fast-food places was changed due to the insistence of the consumers. I also remember a brief time when all the nutritional information was on the tray liner under your food. (Remember, I was a fast-food junkie for a long time.) The reality is that customers didn't like seeing the numbers. Eventually they were moved to a small list hanging on the wall behind the counter—available, but not in your face.

In Brian Wansink's book, *Mindless Eating*, he references a study in which they tested the importance placed by consumers on the availability of nutritional information for the types of food choices they made. They used McDonald's and Subway as their test restaurants for obvious reasons. Subway is now known to the general public as the "healthy chain," and McDonald's, of course, is not. All of Subway's

119

nutritional information is very visible and available. It is listed right next to all of their menu items. The strange outcome was that people ended up eating a higher volume of calories per meal at Subway. Basically, they thought since they were eating healthier they could get a cookie or a bag of chips as well. Overall, they ended up misjudging the calories they consumed by almost 30%. The response for most of the diners at McDonald's was, "I know it is bad for me but it tastes good."[77] So we end up spending our much-needed tax dollars on studies, discussions, and attempts to institute laws meant to sway how people eat without actually telling them what they can and cannot eat. This approach has completely backfired. Developing palates, however, is a method that, in tandem with education about real food, could successfully cultivate a generation of consumers who prefer healthy options, who prefer better options, who, without thinking about it, are supporting a sustainable food system.

This discussion was prompted by concern for the costs associated with health care and the obesity epidemic—all of which are driven by the current budget savings created by the inexpensive food produced in the industrial agricultural system. Though producing more for less with a smaller workforce may have its appeal, the reality is that there is no such thing as cheap food. Maybe you've heard that in some of the local-food marketing press. It might be cheap to produce and cheap to purchase, but the hidden expenses that are directly and indirectly related to making it "cheap" cost us far more in the long run than buying locally and organically. From a restaurant's perspective the initial outlay might be higher, but close examination of the bottom line, once all factors are evaluated, proves we don't save anything, and, in most cases, spend more while trying to cut corners.

PROTECTING THE FARMERS?

An additional commonly cited benefit to industrialized food production is the reduction in labor needed on the farm and the freedom that has afforded other industries to find workers. While our country is more stable as a rule, we are currently facing an unemployment crisis that is not benefited by a decrease in available jobs. In many other countries this is an even direr prospect as farmers are being forced off the farms to live in urban slums and poverty. They are going from growing their own food to looking through garbage to find food.[78] Spinning this as a positive development for the farmers and the farming industry—that they now have the opportunity to leave the farm and get an education, to become a professional—is a dangerous fallacy. When did farming stop being a profession? Farmers, at least all the ones I know, are knowledgeable; even more, they are wise. Truthfully, I find they possess some of the most important knowledge there is to have—information and understanding born out of experience. There is only so much you can learn about farming in the classroom.

The most important education comes through practice, through doing. Every year holds something different, and the rules change. Whether they face lots of rainfall, no rainfall, bugs, poor growing soil, bumper crops, being able to adapt and knowing the land are crucial and come from having experience on a farm. Each farm, each patch of soil, holds its own obstacles and its own solutions. Unfortunately, more and more the farmers aren't leaving by choice. Thousands of farmers throughout the world are losing their farms because the system is set up to put them in debt. What does that mean for us? It means fewer farmers with the know-how and the ability to produce food sustainably and consistently in order to feed our communities. The current food price increase occurring throughout the world is largely connected to the increase in fuel, but it is also connected to large crop failures from the severe weather changes that many countries have experienced in the last few years. Industrial agriculture's by-product is land that, through diversity reduction, loses its ability to withstand severe weather variations.

WHO REALLY BENEFITS?

The last benefit presented was the improved profitability of agricultural companies. This might have been a benefit in the beginning, but has turned into one the biggest causes of the crises for our food system. What was once a large pool of seed companies, fertilizer companies, and pesticide companies has been reduced to just a few companies. Pollan says in *The Omnivore's Dilemma* that there are just four major companies in industrial agriculture. They are well-oiled machines with business success as their primary concern. They are well-connected politically, as many great corporations are in a democratic society. They are global powers with seeds that are literally spread worldwide. You can blame them all you want for the issues we face; but, the fact is we are funding their success, and money talks. Until they are hit at their bottom line they will continue to do business as they are now: profitably.

We need to take another look at the parallels to the tobacco industry. Clearly there is a conflict of interest at play in the decision-making process regarding our food production and the impact on the environment. I will not entirely blame the corporations. They are simply offering a product for us to

122

buy. Ultimately, what we eat or what we buy is our decision. However, it is clear we are not getting all the facts about where our food originates, what goes into it, who is affected by the process, or the lasting impact of their procedures. In researching through books, articles, and documentaries it became very obvious to me that the industry intends to keep us in the dark, and the corporations' refusal to open their doors to cameras or to respond to questions doesn't restore confidence that they are doing the right thing behind their closed doors. It is also obvious that, as a culture, our lack of understanding of the origins of food is not something that is just accepted but desired. It's easy to put the blame on the big companies, and they deserve it, but I would argue that we are equally at fault.

I realize that some of this information may be redundant to those who have followed the same groundbreakers of the local food movement and their dialogue. However, many have not heard this message; and even for those who have, it bears repeating. It is time we all started paying attention, not only to what we eat, but how it's made and how it gets to our plates. But even that is not enough. We have to start demanding and requiring change. As you hopefully see throughout this book, I believe it starts and can be accomplished one kitchen at a time. One chef at a time.

Third tāyst

Chapter Seven
Turning Green

So what??!! Who cares about all of this? By now you're probably thinking: *I understand what you're saying, and I realize that the food system is having some issues. However, my responsibility as a chef is to put out quality food with the lowest food cost in order to maximize profits.* You're probably saying, of course you will buy local, at least a little bit, as long as it doesn't affect the bottom line. I'm sure you know you can get some really high-quality product this way, and, hey, you can jump on the bandwagon of using local food. Then you'll think: *I am already working 70–80 hours a week, why on earth would I want to add more work to my plate? Really, is anybody actually going to be able to tell the difference?* Even if all these statements about the environmental effects of industrial food are true, or even somewhat close to true, can one restaurant make a difference? (Isn't that the typical thought at the start of any revolution?)

These are the basic arguments I get, even from passionate cooks. Although I will say the tide is turning. Now, it seems, if you open a restaurant that is not focused on buying local, or at least marketing that focus, you don't have a chance. It's expected by the public that you are going to use local farmers—an expectation that has become prominent just in the last couple of years. Unfortunately, for the most part, this new reality only affects the independent dining scene. In New York, Chicago, or any other "food" cities where there is a high concentration of foodies (a word as much in need of a definition as *sustainability*), independents seem to be the primary choice for dining. The reality of dining in our country is that, for the majority of the population, the options are limited to chain restaurants and fast-food places. As the restaurant landscape grew over the years, it followed the path of farming and became industrialized. This chain system is not going away, much like fast food is not going away. As we talk about the power of chefs, the corporate chefs in these businesses have a lot of money at their disposal and therefore a lot of power to wield. We need to integrate the positive changes we are discussing into these establishments. A green fast-food chain is a possibility, but maybe we'll need to call it a food-fast restaurant. It focuses on the food first and speed second. It can be done, and it is already starting. Chains such as Chipotle are focusing on greening their operations and showing that sustainable business is smart business. My new sandwich shop Sloco is a great example.

WHY BOTHER?

It's easy to think that one restaurant will not make a difference. I can't really blame those who hold onto these beliefs. For the most part people aren't going to notice if you change your food purchases. They will, however, instantly notice a switch if it's reflected in your menu prices. In these times it is hard to increase prices, as everybody is watching the bottom line. Obviously, after a switch you can print the local farm on the menu, but only a few people will actually notice it. They see filet and stop reading. For those not in the business, this may cause a bit of a stir; but, after almost twenty years of experience, I am positive that people only half-way pay attention to the menu. They see "steak" or "chicken" and a few key words, and that's it. In fact, for those who don't notice the

126

term "grass-finished" on the menu there might even be a few issues regarding the fact that your beef offering is flavorful but a little tough—kind of like the people who order a rib eye and then complain because it is fatty. It happens. All you restaurant folk out there know what I am saying. For example, I had a table once, a deuce, that ordered steaks medium rare. One said it was the best steak ever, the other hated it. Same cow, same loin, cuts from right next to each other, executed (cooked) in the same manner and at the right temperature. By all accounts the steaks were identical. Unfortunately, he wasn't interested in expressing his reasons for disliking the steak, but he disliked it none the less. Somebody probably slapped his dog earlier and he was in a bad mood. That happens. It is easy to allow the lack of public understanding to keep you from making the transition.

If people aren't going to notice the new menu changes, why take the price increase or make the effort, especially in this industry of long hours and low pay? Doesn't this discussion about the lack of acknowledgment completely contradict the newfound local sourcing push? It may seem so, but we have to remember all the food blogs, food noise, and local push are for a very small percentage of the population. When we talk about green restaurants and the power of chefs, we mean making a change for the masses. It's about putting in the extra effort for those who don't necessarily think about the act of eating for pleasure. Most of the time the right way is not necessarily the easy way.

The fact is that one restaurant *will* make a difference. Even a restaurant the size of mine, which feeds approximately 300 people a week, some of them more than once, has the ability to make a big difference in the eyes of the consumer, the community, and the industry. In fact, I know we have made a difference. We were the first restaurant to become certified green in our community and have been extremely fortunate to garner a bit of press regarding this change in our operations. Through that press I feel we have caused a stir locally in how people look at the restaurants they choose. I have been approached by many other restaurant owners and operators questioning the steps I have taken to become green. Is it effective? How much work does it take? How much does it cost? (One of the reasons for writing this book.) Are all these potential customers going to frequent only green restaurants? Are the restaurant owners all going to rush out and get certified as a green place? We may not see radical change immediately, but there is a very good chance that the people who read the press may start questioning the food they purchase and how they operate. If the restaurant owners act on one green step, hopefully one regarding how they purchase food, it is something. Collectively and cumulatively it will make a difference. Previously I mentioned the buying of a little local food with big claims about it, referring to it as "jumping on the bandwagon." If the bandwagon is what it takes, I have no problem with that; even a little bit is a start and a good thing. With the problems we face as a society the reasons for the impetus of change won't matter in the long run. These changes are infectious and, once they start, they spread.

WHY WE DO WHAT WE DO

Something all restaurant folk need to remember is that we are in the service industry and the consumer holds the power. If you need a reason besides social responsibility to buy locally or take some green steps, then know that even in this recession over two-thirds of consumers will make their dining choices based on green issues.[79] It's a good business move. It's quite similar to the industrial food system and the fact that chefs hold the power. Our demands will be met by the companies we support much like we will provide what our customers want.

So far, I have attempted to chart my path in the food world along with the evolution of my understanding of the issues regarding food. I feel it's important to illustrate not only what it takes to be a chef but how the key components of being a successful chef are rooted in knowing how to get good food, being passionate about where your food comes from, and understanding the people who pour themselves into the task of feeding their neighbors. As we continue to evolve in our use of local ingredients, and as that percentage of local ingredients increases, I get more and more comments that encourage us in our efforts. When I hear: "The trout is amazing," or "That broccoli was absolutely delicious, you can taste the freshness," my response is simple. When I get a product that was picked that morning I just try not to screw it up. I can't remember the origin of the statement, but I vividly remember hearing that a chef's skill lies not in his ability to make good food flavorful—because it already is flavorful—but it is in the chef's ability to coerce flavors out of food that doesn't have flavor to begin with. That comment, to me, was indicative of how our food supply has deteriorated. For a squash or tomato to be devoid of flavor is inconceivable, but, sadly, true. The fact that a typical ingredient travels nearly 1,500 miles before it reaches your plate means there are now tomatoes, and many other products, genetically modified to be "perfect" and last forever. Environmental issues aside, how can we as a society be okay with continuing the use of a food system that produces flavorless food? At least until we process it with our wonderful flavor crystals or whatever the industries use. Do we really want to end up as a society that pops a breakfast, lunch, and dinner calorie pill?

This passion that drives me to make the best food I can is what led me to the practice of sourcing local product. Knowing my local product opened my eyes to the connection of our food to us, our health, our communities, and our children's futures . . . to *my* children's futures.

I have tried to show the connection between the growth of our food and the environment, the state of our communities, and our health because these connections are the reasons I took my restaurant and my life green. My children were the other reason. For me going green was a direct result of understanding what it takes to grow food for a thriving, healthy population, now and in the future. Food is the one unifying element between the people of the world. Everyone has to eat to live. If the ability to grow food falters in any one area or a once prolific growing region ceases to be so, it will have a negative rippling effect the world over.

There are many reasons for this, one being the globalization of our economy, our commerce, and our communications. As Americans, we typically will not sit idly by while another country starves or is in jeopardy.

We will try to help—send financial or military aid, food, etc. We have a vested interest in the survival of the global community. The environmental impacts we have been discussing are another reason for thinking beyond our local needs. However, it is also a result of the industrialized system we have developed—the transformation of food into a commodity, combined with the decreasing resources of the planet—that has had a staggering ripple effect on the state of the planet. A food system that needs to take in more "calories" than it can produce is one that cannot continue indefinitely. It cannot be sustainable. So as we push forward with this system that is, according to its proponents, the only answer to feeding the increasing population of the world, we must consider the actual cost to our planet as a whole. We combine forces with countries willing to help each other to end hunger; yet we still have almost half the population on the planet facing food-related battles from one end of the spectrum—hunger and malnutrition—to the other—obesity and diet-related diseases. The web of the food system and the damage that the wrong system can cause is complicated and requires a unified effort. However, I find encouragement in knowing what the right system can accomplish. In restaurants, food is definitely the biggest factor they can contribute to creating a sustainable industry, but it is still only a part of the impact a restaurant has on the system.

I am involved in some organizations that gather with the purpose of advancing a sustainable food system and educating chefs to further that goal. Last year I was at a conference with other like minded industry people and I was taken aback at the—for lack of a better term—disdain I encountered over my green certification. After a couple of days, I flat out asked one of the board members about what I was observing. I was sensing this animosity from the majority of the people at this conference. My feeling was right. There was, of course, some history and politics involved, which is understandable; but, I was still shocked that these individuals, so focused on a sustainable food system, seemed so indifferent about the importance of a green restaurant. How can you focus on one and not the other? It's hypocritical to swear by your passion for sustainable sourcing and not pay attention to the amount of waste you generate, to the efforts for water conservation, or any of the hundreds of other ways restaurants can improve operations. We might not be able to avoid shady business people, and "greenwashing" will be an issue until being green becomes standard. In case you are unfamiliar, "greenwashing: is the use of green marketing or the claiming of green business practices without actually doing so. But I will stand by my earlier statement that even if restaurants start for the wrong reasons, at least they've started. That being said, for individuals who are leaders in the sustainable food movement not to look at the effects of the industry as a whole, in my opinion, is worse than greenwashing. It was probably political and maybe there was more behind-the-scenes stuff. Who knows? But I don't believe politics or personal history should stand in the way of any improvements someone wants to make. For that matter, maybe they really do believe in this idea of green restaurants, but it didn't come off that way.

Even in light of that eye opening experience, I am glad to report that the momentum the food movement has right now is incredible. That conference, the organization, and what they are achieving is amazing. The previous story is relevant because the importance of greening the restaurant beyond the food is still way down the list in the fight for sustainability. If we are truly talking about a sustainable food system, then the businesses that utilize half the sustainable product need to be sustainable in their operations as well.

The positive result from my experience at that conference and the discussion also made me realize the importance of focusing on the restaurant as a whole. We were already doing that, but had yet to verbally acknowledge its importance. Michael Pollan talks about the need to have a holistic approach to eating in order to be truly healthy. Sustainable food activists talk as much about the importance of a regenerative food system with decreased waste and energy use being just as important as decreased antibiotic use. They focus on the system as a whole. The restaurant industry needs to do the same.

I constantly tell people that when I made this decision it was the result of an evolution stemming from my newfound understanding of the connectivity of the food system; as a chef-driven restaurant, I cannot be this passionate about sourcing food the right way and not push that focus to the front of the house. How can any restaurant claiming to be focused on sustainability in the kitchen not apply that philosophy to their operations? How can you not look at sustainability in restaurants universally?

Sustainable food and green business practices go hand in hand. Buying local is important, but so are practices such as switching light bulbs, recycling, and using unbleached parchment. The logic for both is the same, and for these reasons we went green.

Chapter Eight
Assessment

Once you have decided to take the plunge into the right way to do business (yes, this sounds arrogant, but it *is* all about making money), when you consider the "triple bottom line"—social, economic, and ecological—rather than just the economic bottom line, you will see it is the better way to run your operations. Sustainable practices will make you more money in the long run.

From this decision your next step will be to determine a path. You can go it alone. You can forge ahead with personal research and Internet answers. You can look for companies or consultants to help you. More and more are popping up, some with the right motivations, and some just interested in capitalizing on a trend. (I would stay away from the companies that offer green assistance [with or without certification] connected to existing companies who also carry a full line of the products required for you to be green.) Or, you can seek third-party certification—companies like the Green Restaurant Association (GRA), who offer assistance and certification for a fee; but they also offer, as far as I can tell, the best assurance to customers looking for validation. Customer validation is the purpose for a certification. It provides you with proof against the naysayers and individuals who think it's all a waste of time and money—thus, the reason to stay away from the companies offering a for-profit certification while simultaneously selling the green products required. If a certification is for validation, then a certification from a company selling you product is less validating in the eyes of the skeptic.

Regardless of the path you choose, the next stage of operational change is to assess your current environmental footprint. The assessment will provide you with a baseline understanding of your operations, allowing you to move forward.

GETTING STARTED

Have you ever thought about starting at the front of your property and going over every inch from one side to the other and from the front to the back? Well, for me it was as overwhelming as it sounds. I can't imagine what it would be like for someone with a big restaurant. Still, after the two to three days that my sous chef and I took filling out our assessment worksheet, I did find it somewhat rewarding. It is amazing what you learn about your operations when you look at them from a different angle, one of energy use and waste management rather than cleanliness and organization. It also forces you to think about how many seemingly insignificant functions you take for granted that actually have serious cost and/or environmental impacts. Have you ever really looked at the costs per kilowatt of electricity or per gallon of water on your monthly bill? The restaurant business is a business of pennies, but until I started the greening process I had only looked at non-food bills as a whole. What were my total utilities for the year? It wasn't that we didn't try to be conscientious about shutting off the water and turning off the lights, but it also wasn't something at the forefront of our minds. I never thought about breaking these costs down to their individual elements. It's kind of ironic when you consider that in the kitchen everything is broken down into ounces to determine prices. Again, why would you not replicate that practice everywhere? It's easy to justify inaction by saying there is just not enough time to do everything you need to do without adding more to the plate. The truth is, this is an unbelievably beneficial exercise and I recommend all restaurant folk take the time to assess their business from an environmental point of view. The information you gather is highly enlightening, and if applied to your practices, will most likely result in an improved bottom line.

Parking Lots and Pavement

So where do you start? Like I said, you start at one end of the property and systematically move to the other. Starting outside, some of the questions you'll have to answer are: How many parking spots are there? Is it pre-marked or free parking? Are there preferred spots for green cars, bike racks, etc.? What type of paving material? Are you in a leased building on a property sharing a parking lot with another building? Is it asphalt, pretty much like every parking lot in the city? Remember, I was just starting out doing this whole green thing, and I didn't have much information, particularly about how many connections there are between the various layers of business operations and how they're interrelated. My thoughts were running amok: *Why the hell does the parking lot matter? What restaurant doesn't have a parking lot? How many surfacing options can there be?* Well, it turns out that impermeable surfaces like our asphalt parking lot, or concrete (like our porch), blacktop, etc., have some pretty significant effects.

To keep it short and sweet, the problem is in the name. They are impermeable surfaces, primarily to water. It rains, and the water runs over them collecting all of these

137

wonderful extras along the way—stuff like garbage, pesticides, and toxic metals leftover from tires. Where does all of this crap end up? Not in treatment plants but in our waterways. The majority of storm water is not treated in the municipal plants. Only when it is mixed with sewage will the water run through a municipal treatment plant and on high-flow days there is a good chance that raw sewage is escaping into our streams. According to the U.S. Environmental Protection Agency (EPA), storm-water runoff is credited with 21% of lake and 45% of stream pollution. So really, the only concern is when the flow gets too intense for the treatment plants to handle, which also happens to be a major by-product of impermeable paving. If you are one of those who are anti-green, this is a bunch of crap hoopla, people, then look at it in a purely self-serving manner. In areas with large amounts of pavement, such as in heavily populated cities, the constant runoff from asphalt is perpetuating this storm-water pollution problem. The increased square footage of pavement also prevents water from absorbing into the ground, thereby decreasing the water table, causing the available potable water to decrease. Translation: Your access to clean water is affected. This is a perfect example of the domino effect of environmental damage.

The fact is that there are porous surfacing methods that have been around since the 1970s. As with most green building innovations, initial cost has been the biggest hindrance in these methods being used more frequently. Yet it is another great example of how the green way is often the better business move. The permeable paving solutions maximize groundwater recharge, lessen downstream flooding, and stream-bank erosion. They also decrease production costs by eliminating the need for drainage and retention systems, which additionally reduces the cost of compliance with storm-water regulatory requirements.[80] But these techniques are not used as often as they should be because they are more expensive. In a direct cost comparison of pouring pavement versus laying a permeable surface, permeable types of paving are more expensive. However, in the long run, these environmentally friendly techniques will save you on your overall costs. In Nashville, we have seen water costs increase over the past few years due to necessary cleanup in the stormwater system. It sounds quite similar to the "cheap" food discussion doesn't it? Paving appears to be the cheaper way to go, but if you take into account all the residual costs, such as waterways cleanup and resulting pollution cleanup, that number changes dramatically. These costs will find their way back to your pocket.

Outside-In

So far, we have made it about three inches into our assessment. Next up was the description of the landscaping on our property with exact measurements and the percentage of plants in the soil. Ours is kind of small, about 8 feet by 15 feet, and includes only two plants with some seasonal herbs taking up just shy of 50% of the space—pretty minimal in my eyes, but relevant in the grand scheme of things. Next, what type of building is it? What are the construction materials? How many square feet? Are there sidewalks?

After the external structural evaluation, we started looking at waste and recycling because those containers were outside. At the time we only recycled cardboard. We share a dumpster and the cardboard recycling with our landlord and at a pretty reasonable rate compared to other restaurants' waste costs, although it, too, has gone up significantly in the last

139

couple of years. My landlord is also kind of particular on how things are handled, so digging around in the existing company to find out about possible recycling options had to be handled gently. We did not recycle any other products because it is not a requirement of the city, and they do not pick up commercial recycle containers. (Chapter 14, "Waste and Recycling," will cover the steps we took to change this practice.) To finish outside we had to provide information on our grease trap and grease disposal methods.

Power and Heat and Water, Oh My!

At this point, we finally turned our attention to the utilities and how much of them we used. We had to calculate exactly how much we used per year and then break it down to a monthly average. We then had to break it down further to get the cost per unit. This is one of those times when we looked at what we were spending and realized how easy it would be to cut back a little here or a little there and lower costs. These were savings that would go directly to the bottom line. As a restaurateur or a chef you are always (or should always) be looking for any way to cut costs. We started with electricity. The restaurant industry is the largest consumer of electricity in the retail sector, using close to five times more than the next closest industry. It equals almost one-third of all energy used by the retail sector. To add to that, 93% of the electricity in the United States is made from polluting nonrenewable resources.[81] We used about 10,247.37 kilowatts per month and were charged .08634 cents per kilowatt. Obviously this is an average and can fluctuate significantly. We did this assessment in late winter/early spring of 2008 using numbers from 2007. We averaged around $850 per month on our electric bill. Just after this assessment the cost of utilities started to rise. Our average cost for 2010 was around $1,000 per month even though we have decreased our energy usage by almost 25%. So we are using much less and paying much more. I shudder to think what my costs would be without the changes! Well . . . I guess they would be 25% more, so about $250 a month or $3,000 per year. That is a pretty significant savings.

Lighting Up the Place

Sometimes, throughout this process, you get a little comic relief—unexpected reminders of how new some of this stuff is to most people. For example, the occupancy sensors for light switches, which are a very fiscally doable change, are not a new product, but people don't expect to see them in a restaurant. I haven't researched exactly how long they have been around, but I have to say it is kind of fun watching people's reactions. (Note: I am not hanging out in the bathrooms just to see people's reactions, but it is really fun to catch a glimpse of them entering the bathroom for the first time.) People are not used to going into a bathroom in a restaurant in the dark. We have strategically placed our sensors in a location so they turn on when the door is opened. Still, it can take a couple of seconds to respond. I want to point out how important it is to figure out what is the most "strategic location." We really thought about where to place them for ideal use. We measured movements, light refraction, all the potential situations for most effective performance . . . Not really. We actually just put them right where the original switches were. We didn't have the money or the time for anything else. Now the time it takes for the light to come on is not really that long at first glance; but, when you think about it (count one Mississippi, two

Mississippi . . .), it would feel awkward standing in an unfamiliar bathroom with no light even for a fraction of a second. In fact, in the men's room, we discovered the rubber cover over the sensor was pushed in after about a week. I tried to replicate that move on another sensor just to see what it would take to permanently indent the cover and it wasn't easy. Whoever did it really wanted that light to go on or off. It just goes to show you how unfamiliar people are with some of the green innovations. I won't even go into the dual flush toilet stories.

Cooking with Gas

Gas was next, and, unfortunately, in a standard restaurant it is a hard place to really conserve. We were using about 492.75 thermal units a month and paying 1.2552 cents per thermal unit. We have two months in which we use gas heat, then the only other uses are the cooking equipment and the water heaters. I had no idea how much gas a standard water heater used. They heat from the bottom requiring significant time for the water to reach the proper temperature; the bigger the tank, the longer the process. Add to that the basic physics of hot rising and cold sinking and it is a long process. They are basically giant stock pots that are constantly simmering, essentially wasting gas. My thermal use is relatively low, except for those two months, and it is nearly impossible to cut back on what we use for cooking.

Rinse Cycle

Water is the last utility we evaluated. Water makes the world go around. It is more important than money, and in this global

142

marketplace of diminishing resources and water shortages, water is traded in a similar fashion. It is no different for restaurants. They cannot legally open their doors without water—water for cooking, water for washing, water to drink, water to thaw, water for the bathrooms, water for ice, water to cool, water for steam. Water, in Nashville, is the least expensive of all the utilities at .0094 cents per gallon right now. This is up from .0081 cents last year and went up again recently after an increase in storm water and sewage treatment. But it is amazing how much water is wasted in a day. We used, at the time of our assessment, 50–60 CCF per month. That is, on average, 40,000 gallons of water a month. Looking at that number makes me wonder how the GRA's quoted average of 300,000 gallons per year is accurate. We are only open five nights a week, and were using almost 500,000 gallons per year.

Open Spaces

While we were in the office/wine storage/equipment storage/desks and file cabinets area figuring out the utility breakdowns, we decided to start the inside facility assessment. We had to count the type and number of lights. We recorded each type of paper we used, and its make and model. We looked at the energy efficiency of all our equipment: the type of computer, fax, phone system, as well as the types of power strips and how many of each. By this point, it was getting tedious, and in my restaurant the office is right next to the front door. We had literally traveled no more than fifteen feet since we started.

Next up, the bar. How many seats? Check the sink and the gallons per minute (GPM) of the faucet. What is the make and model of the dishwasher? Do you have any coolers and what are their make and model? I think by now you get the idea. This detail-by-detail assessment continued throughout the whole restaurant.

We listed all the coolers with their specifications. We noted the number and types of air conditioners/heaters. We included the ice machine and the walk-in, specifying size. We looked at the thermostats used to control the air, and the number of fans or ventilation exits for the A/C (that would be twenty-seven, by the way). We counted and measured the windows. We included the make and model of the water heater and the hood. Then we got into our linens. What types of napkins and how many did we go through? Ditto on the tablecloths and bar towels. We listed the toilet paper, the roll towels, the c-folds, the disposable toilet seat covers. We don't really have those, but it was on the list. We had to look at the lighting inside and out—from the office to the bathrooms, through the dining room, the kitchen, the server area, the walk-in, and so on. What type was our ceiling and did it have insulation? If so, what was the type of insulation? Don't forget about cleaning products. How many, what type? If you're a new restaurant, there is another list entirely for the build-out that breaks down all the building supplies, waste control, paint, artwork, etc.

What's Cookin?

Finally the assessment came to an end with a look into the kitchen, into the heart of mine (or any restaurant) and the impetus for this green assessment. Where did our food come from, and what were the percentage breakdowns of where we got it (i.e., organic, local, vegetarian, or vegan, and sustainable seafood)? We finished with a comprehensive list of our

144

vendors plus their accompanying invoices. Don't let the brevity of this kitchen assessment paragraph fool you. It was an intensive task. However, we have focused so much on the food up to this point you should have a good idea of the assessment focus.

It was an overwhelming task. Yet it was also very fulfilling. It is easy to become complacent in the daily grind, and when you're in the restaurant business you live in the business day in and day out. You spend more time at the restaurant than at your home. I think it is easy to become oblivious to your surroundings. Things begin to blend in and you look right over them. Taking the time to go through and complete this assessment is something that should be done every couple of years. Granted, equipment doesn't change that frequently, but you can definitely build on the original assessment. Use the information to track your cost-cutting moves. Take the time, even though there is never enough, and do this assessment. Obviously, I think it should be a start to the greening of your restaurant; but, even if you choose not to follow that path, you can use it to save money and improve your bottom line. It was the start of a long journey for us. It was a taste of what going green, and more importantly, being certified green was going to be like. This was a big cliff and we had just jumped.

For information on GRA certification visit their website: http://www.dinegreen.com/restaurants/standards.asp.

Chapter Nine
Evaluation

After the assessment is complete it's time for the evaluation. If you're getting assistance this is a hurry–up-and-wait situation. When it came to our assessment evaluation I wanted answers immediately, I wanted to make decisions and I wanted to go for it. Maybe it's due to years of being in the kitchen and having to make snap decisions. Regardless of what made me this way, I tend to go for it, to try it and see what happens. If it doesn't work, I'll try something else but at least I tried it and found out it wasn't the right (or most effective) move. This philosophy will work for most small things, themed wine dinners, special events, happy hours, etc.; but, when it comes to making a major change, I don't make quick decisions at all, like this decision to go green. This process afforded me a great lesson as well. I learned to discern when to make a quick decision and when to take the time to analyze the options.

We've found ourselves at a crossroads, faced with a big decision: What is our next move? What steps do we take? How do we implement them? These are the same kinds of questions you'll have to answer after your assessment. For *tāyst*, a small business with almost no funds, we had to be very careful to do this as strategically as possible, calculating how it would play into our everyday business and cash flow.

I've commented before that if you have a pocketful of money, it is much easier to make green changes, and that is true to an extent. But "easier" is really relative to the situation. It is easier when you are trying to figure out whether to put film on the windows or replace your air conditioner. An energy saver A/C unit is more expensive, but it will conserve more energy and save money in the long run. Window films will help to control temperature fluctuation to a small extent. One will cost thousands, the other a couple of hundred. Ideally, having both is the best answer. If money is not an issue and you only want to do one, the A/C unit will typically yield the most noticeable results. It's a personal decision and the answer will be different for everyone. Behavioral changes are not any easier—a new waste program, for example—because now you are not talking about just switching a cooler but about changing the habits of your employees and yourself. So that begs the question: What is the best way to change?

Maybe my passion for food is somewhat blinding, but everything circles back to food in some way or another for me. There is no absolute right answer. Every place is different, and every chef/restaurant should follow their own path. Is every single farm run exactly the same way (please exclude the industrial operations)? Is every carrot grown in exactly the same fashion as the season before? How many chefs have you worked for and how differently do they operate? The type of business might be the same, but each one has a little different touch or feel to it. It's another part of human nature. It's impossible to give you an exact blueprint for how to make a restaurant green; the plan has to fit the place. It needs to be individualized for it to be successful.

WHERE DO WE GO FROM HERE?

After my assessment was finished and sent to my consultant at the GRA, we waited, and waited, and waited. Okay, it wasn't really that long, but it felt that way to me. I had been in constant conversation with my consultant for the entire process up to this point so I had a good idea of where to start. The normal timeline for the certification process—from assessment to certification—was about four months. We signed the contract and completed our assessment in the middle of February, and it was my hope to be certified by Earth Day. So I went ahead and started figuring out some changes for myself. My consultant was very knowledgeable and I was paying her to guide me, but I just felt the need to power forward on my own. It's also one of the reasons I know what I know today.

The way the certification process worked at that time was relatively simple, but it has changed quite a bit since I went through it. At that time, a restaurant was required to make four improvements to their operations each year. This was relatively easy in the beginning; but, I got the sense that, as the years go by, it would become increasingly difficult. In the back of my mind, and with my "outside voice" for that matter, I questioned being able to continually make this kind of progress each year. When I questioned the feasibility of making four changes a year, the response from the GRA was: *You can always be greener.* They were right. There is always a better way to go, an improvement you can make, and new technology for approaching a zero carbon footprint. To truly reach that state is, at this time, almost impossible. But none of this is about being perfect. It is about constantly improving your operations along with like-minded others who will eventually make the difference. Isn't that how we should work anyway? Shouldn't every chef always be building on what they have done previously? Shouldn't we always try to be and do better?

The first two steps were required—the elimination of all Styrofoam in the building and the start of a recycling

148

program that was compliant with the local government. Getting rid of Styrofoam would be relatively easy, or so I thought. We would just purchase some biodegradable to-go containers. As we have found out in every step that we have done, there are no easy answers. Today, green take-away products can be found virtually everywhere; but, at the time we were looking, my normal avenues of procurement didn't even supply an option for something that was just a "greener" product than the rest. It is, however, a great example of the positive direction the industry is going. The second step didn't sit well with me. Our local government didn't have any policies on commercial recycling, unless you count their lack of a policy—meaning, they offered no programs, no service, and no direction. There were some sites around the city set up as recycling centers, but that was an unrealistic option. We could have just continued with our cardboard program, and it would have been enough for certification. As I said, that wasn't good enough for us, so we went out and found our own company to pick up our recycling. Interestingly enough, this company was just starting out as well.

Two steps down, two to go. After looking at the assessment and recognizing that almost everything we did from an operational standpoint needed to be changed, we decided to make a combination of large and small changes. The decisions we made were based on a number of factors: cost, time, functionality, GRA requirements, and the size of our business.

CH-CH-CH-CHANGES!

Every single step you take has a price attached to it. Even behavioral changes such as pulling your frozen product a day before you need it to avoid using running water for thawing will cost you an extra ten minutes of labor at the end of the night. Each step has a cost-benefit analysis to be performed. The cost may be as small as $1 for water aerators or it may be as expensive as $5,000–$10,000 for an Energy Star air conditioner. I am not saying you need to bring in a consulting firm to lay out your future, but you need to look at the pros and cons of each step from a business standpoint as well as an ecological one. The cost must also be viewed in terms of initial outlay and long-term benefits rather than as purely an immediate expense. Obviously, the immediate hit still plays a part because you need to have cash flow in order to make a purchase such as an air conditioner; but, if the money is there, you need to ask yourself how much that Energy Star–rated system will save you in the long run. Simply factor in the percentage of energy and water used by the A/C units now—typically about 28% of water use and about 17% of energy use—and compare it to the increased cost of the unit.[82] Currently, we have an air conditioner that I have to caress and love to keep it working through the summers. I have already replaced one of the systems in the main dining room. Unfortunately, it was before we went green and I stupidly didn't get an Energy Star system. I wish I knew then what I know now because it would have been well worth the difference in price. For instance, these Energy Star systems run $1,000 to $2,000 more than a regular system, potentially around $4,000, depending on the size. (This price difference is based on some estimates that I have already received for the soon-to-be-replaced unit.) Based on my water bill averaging $300 a month and my electric bill averaging $1,000 per month, I could potentially save almost $960 a year in combined water and electric savings, according to the EPA's estimates that a

150

30% reduction in cooling costs occurs with an Energy Star-rated system.[83] Now, in reality, it will probably not be a total drop of that percentage so my savings will probably end up between $750 and $900 per year. Regardless, the Energy Star unit has paid for the added cost in one to two years, and then you will continue to receive the added benefit of the savings each year after that. Factor into the equation the trend of increasing utility bills, and your savings will be even higher.

What to Consider

There are a few factors to consider in this process. The cost definitely comes into play at two major times in the greening of a restaurant—during the opening and when equipment is replaced. Let's face it, we are not to going to buy new equipment if the old equipment is working fine. Only when a piece of equipment goes down will we be faced with the decision to spend more for the green choice or just replace it with a similar non-environmental unit. That can only be determined by your cash flow situation. If you can afford to go green at that time, it is definitely in your best interests to do so. You will add dollars to the bottom line and be environmentally friendly at the same time.

The next factor is time. We were under a self-imposed time crunch. This probably will not be the case for most people. When we decided on our steps I purposely looked for the low hanging fruit, for the modifications we could accomplish quickly. Light bulbs are a great example of this. Here is a quick and easy way to cut 75% of your energy usage related to lighting: switch to compact fluorescent lamps (CFL). However, the CFLs are not the only option, and switching to them is not as easy as buying squiggly light bulbs.

Unfortunately, what should have been an easy change was anything but. We eventually changed our bulbs after ten months of research and trial and error. Not all steps will require this much time. If you are open seven days a week, it may be hard to find a day to shut down and replace a unit or your windows, etc., and in the restaurant world, time is measured in seconds.

Another factor—functionality—also plays a part in your decisions, especially when you are talking about behavioral changes. Waste, again, would be the best example of this. How you dispose of waste is less a financial issue (although that will play a part) and more a personnel issue. They go from tossing everything into the same can, or multiple cans, placed throughout the restaurant, to separating all the trash into a variety of specific cans. The longer you've been open, the more effort this will take. Trash cans are moved, decreased in number, signs and labels are put up, all in order to aid the staff in following the new procedures. No longer can you blindly toss your trash in whichever can is closest. Food waste goes into compost, plastic and metal go into recycling, foil and plastic wrap are put into regular trash. You go from five trash cans in the kitchen to one trash, one recycle, and one compost can. Just to make things fun, glass is totally separate and no longer in the kitchen at all. Or do you, instead, look at window films, which can cut down on your electric costs by helping to control the temperature of your room? What will it take to hang them, and will they stay on? I can report, for us, after about a year and a half, they are still on and seem to be effective; although, since they were implemented at the same time as other energy-saving techniques, I can't give you hard numbers from our experience.

One of the last factors when determining your steps is the size of your business. I am fortunate in that I have a small restaurant with one staff—meaning everybody works every shift. One of the benefits of a staff like this is the cohesiveness which develops over time. Although each is different in their personalities, we work with the same mindset. Everyone who works for me, in the front and back of the house, has the same type of passion for the food we serve. Through that passion for food they also have a passion for the state of the environment. Or, maybe their passion for the environment makes them passionate about our food. Regardless, they are aware of the connection between the two and are totally behind the moves we are making to lessen our footprint. It's been a long time since I worked in a large operation so it would be hard to say from experience how these changes could affect a larger staff.

According to other members of the GRA, going green seriously improves staff morale. I would definitely agree with that assessment, but more importantly, going green increases your business, which also boosts the morale of your staff by putting more money in their pockets. Once again we come back to the financial motivation for going green! Regardless of the reason, increased morale is a good thing for your business. Happy employees make happy customers. The only potential issues I can see regarding the size of your business are similar to those affecting functionality. Certain behavioral changes might be easier with a smaller staff than a larger one, which may play a role in how you choose your steps. With a larger staff, it might be smarter to start with less complicated action points to help change the mind-set of the staff before moving to the bigger behavioral changes. Individuals who believe in a cause are more likely to put the effort into making that cause successful, even if it means extra work.

THE RESULTS ARE IN

All of these factors played a part in the decisions we made regarding our assessment. When our evaluation came back, it suggested five options for us to choose from. These options were suggested with our consultant's knowledge of our particular situation: no money. This is the benefit of using a third party with a consultant—personal understanding and directional help. We were given a list of steps from the GRA with details about what we were doing and its environmental impact. It looked something like this:

- Establish a Glass Recycling Program—I had found a company to take glass, which would divert waste from landfills and incinerators as well as supply material for post-consumer recycled products. Recycled products reduce demand for extracting natural resources from the environment. It saves natural resources, energy, landfill space, and reduces pollution by avoiding mining or harvesting of virgin materials.[84]

- Eliminate Styrofoam Containers—We would switch to a recyclable or biodegradable to-go container. By doing this, we would be protecting human health and the environment from the harmful effects of styrene.[85]

- Switch All Paper to 100% PCW Recycled Paper—Recycled paper is one of the most flexible green moves out there, with a lot of variation in the options. The best option is 100% post-consumer waste (PCW) paper. This means that 100% of the paper was made from products that are being reused. When the paper is listed as 30%

it means that 30% is reused material, but the rest can be, and typically is, virgin trees. The other type of recycled paper is listed as "made from R.P.," post-industrial, pre-consumer, or recovered. This paper is left over from the paper-making process and is usually blended with virgin paper. "Every ton of 100% post-consumer waste recycled paper products you buy saves 12 trees, 1,196 gallons of water, 1,087 pounds of solid waste, 3 cubic yards of landfill space, 1,560 kilowatts of energy, 1,976 lbs. of greenhouse gases and 390 gallons of oil (29)."[86]

- Add Aerators to Faucets to Conserve Water—To do this we would purchase .5 gpm (gallons through the faucet in a minute) for all sinks except the triple compartment in the kitchen on which we could use 1.5 gpm aerators. Can you say pissed-off cooks? The hand sinks in the bathrooms and server areas were an easy transition, but the decrease from a 2.2 gpm to a 1.5 gpm in the kitchen almost caused a mutiny. (Remember that comment about restaurants running on seconds? Nowhere is that more true than in the kitchen. When you need something, you need it yesterday because there is always more work to do than there is time to do it.) By adding time to the prep by decreasing the amount of water coming through the faucet, you end up with unhappy cooks. At least until they get used to it . . : I'll let you know when that happens. The established cooks are fine, but it drives new-hires crazy. The good news about these aerators is that they are the easiest, most affordable, and one of the most effective changes you can make. I would suggest, actually urge, everyone to get these for their homes and definitely for their restaurants, especially when you consider the average water use for a restaurant. They cost about a dollar apiece, give or take a few cents. Since I have put them on my faucets we have averaged a savings of 14,000 gallons of water per month. They amount to about a 25–30% reduction in water usage. Add the "behavioral" form of water conservation to that, maybe some Energy Star equipment, and you are potentially looking at a 50% decrease in water usage.

- Purchase 40% PCW To-Go Bags—I am kind of an overachiever, so we did more steps than were required or recommended. We didn't actually take credit for the menu paper step in our original certification that we had already taken. For some time I had been investigating the potential use of beeswax candles, so we chose to go with the candles instead of the menu paper (that story to follow). It was a time-related decision on our part. I had the candles ready to go and the paper was going to take a little longer, and I wanted to get certified by Earth Day.

That is the way the evaluation worked for us. It seems really compacted and not that big a deal when I look at it recorded on these pages; but, while it was happening, it was pretty intense. I was still cooking, doing the accounting, and running the restaurant, yet somehow found the time to squeeze this in. I was 100% invested in the right way to start running my business. That is key. We talked about "greenwashing" and "bandwagon local" and the need to acknowledge that even a little bit is a start. But if you're going to make the green leap, you must be 100% behind it in the beginning or it won't get the attention it needs. It will fall by the wayside as time demands take you in other directions. But if you are totally committed, it will quickly become second nature.

STARTING OVER

In the beginning of 2009 the GRA changed the way in which they certify, and every restaurant with a previous certification would have to start over again. The actions taken up to this point would count, but the system used to judge the restaurants was completely changed. You might be wondering why I chose to spend the time describing the initial certification process if it is out of date. First, I think the impact of change can be better sensed through first-hand experiences. By reading the stories of my changes I feel you can better grasp what it might be for you. Second, there was a very real criticism of this initial method, the lack of requirements for food. That being said, with the yearly need for continuous change, food would eventually have to be addressed, but in the beginning, certification could be achieved without sustainable food. In the restaurant industry, food has to be the driving force. However, as we have established, it was a start, and without that we would not be experiencing the push for green restaurants as we are now.

I am not going to say I wasn't frustrated when this new system was announced. After all, I had just finished the process with the first certification. Once I let the new system sink in, I realized the importance of the implemented changes. A full description and breakdown of the requirements is in Appendix B, but I will include a quick breakdown here.

The GRA moved from a step-based system to a point system. Throughout the operation, each type of material, equipment, and procedure was giving a point value. By breaking down the restaurant in this manner, they leveled the playing field across the country. It also started to focus more on the restaurant as a whole. In order to achieve certification you now had to amass a total number of points, 100 for a two-star certification, 175 for a 3-star certification, and 300 for a four-star certification. (Currently there is only one four-star green restaurant in the country.) The points were broken into various categories: water, energy, food, disposables, chemicals, build-out, and waste, with a minimum point total required in all categories for certification to be given.

I must say that, although I do like the new system and understand its importance in leveling the playing field, I don't think the food criteria represent the percentages accurately. The current breakdown is based on the percentage of dollars spent on food that is local, organic, grass-fed, certain number of miles to restaurant, etc. Basing these points on the cost of food versus the total amount used is the only potential way to measure food points, but, at least for me, it cuts down on the percentage of sustainable product that we actually use. For example, we have one or two fish items on the menu, but they account for 25% of my dollars spent on food. They have a much higher cost per pound than my nose-to-tail pork, lamb, or beef. So, pound-for-pound, the cost representation is skewed even though it's one or two dishes out of twenty. It may seem nit-picky because the point scale is the same for everyone, but it does affect my rating.

All-in-all, the new point system is a much more effective way to evaluate restaurant practices. It is a holistic representation, which is of utmost importance. Once you go through the assessment and evaluation process, you will have a much better picture of where you are, where you want to be, and how to get there.

Chapter Ten
Groundwork

So you've made the decision to dive in. You've either chosen to go with a certification or to go it alone, you've evaluated your operation, and you've assessed the areas on which you need to focus. It's time to start building the foundation for your changes and transform your restaurant or your concept into one that is ecologically responsible. You are ready to operate a business that is focused on the "triple bottom line," a green restaurant.

After spending two-plus years writing this book, things obviously have changed. The search for the sustainable way is now second nature for us, and, yet, some changes are still a battle. When I started writing this book we had been certified for about a year. After digging ourselves into the process, you would think that the excitement had waned. But to this day we still get excited about things. Whenever you do anything that will make a difference, it is exciting. Whenever you overcome a challenge, even one as simple as finding a consistent source for organic sugar, it's exciting. I don't think that will ever go away. I certainly hope it never goes away. Is it shocking that I would relate it to food? Every new dish brings excitement and reignites the passion. When a thought becomes reality, it's the completion of the journey to bring that idea to fruition. It may not happen the way you envision it, but once you achieve your goal, big or small, it's thrilling. The anticipation as these changes start to fall into place can be overwhelming. The hardest part will be fighting the desire to change everything at once. Remember: This lifestyle is infectious. You will need to proceed with a controlled plan.

The easiest way to take restaurants green is to start at the beginning. Raise more start-up funds and pay the extra for the Energy Star equipment. Put in solar panels if you can. Include the double-pane windows and all the fixin's and watch your savings come down the road. I realize that it is easier to write it than to do it, but your efforts will pay off in the long run. Establish the behavior protocols from the first day. If that is your reality, fantastic! For all the other restaurants out there, like mine, who need to make changes to an existing operation, it is a puzzle to solve.

A MEASURED APPROACH

When you are looking at your evaluation try to step back and look at all the areas in which you need to make changes. Break down all the factors related to their implementation. Weigh the costs and benefits of each. Take the time to think about the most effective way to proceed, one that will decrease cash flow disruption as much as possible. Change starts with an in-depth cost-benefit analysis of all the potential steps and resulting expenditures.

This is also the time to think about some actions you might never think possible. It can't hurt to reach for what may seem to be unreachable goals. To have these goals on the horizon from the beginning of your changes increases the possibility that they may occur. Conversely, you need to pay attention to all the *little* changes that are possible as well. Make a list or a spreadsheet or some format that works for you. Put everything on it. Break the list down with a mix of choices that are inexpensive, expensive with a good payback, and more expensive but very environmentally friendly with the cost spread out over time. Also include in that list the environmental benefits that are gained by implementing each change. We are, after all, talking about integrating an ecologically responsible focus into the business decisions. The environmental benefit comes into play as much if not more than the finances.

Once your spreadsheet or chosen format is done, lay out the time frame in which you want to proceed. Make sure you give yourself ample time. Don't rush it and make the wrong move. I was fortunate in that my initial changes were all very beneficial. It very easily could have gone the other direction. In my haste to get certified I could have spent too much cash on the wrong step, seriously affecting the business. Just as when you are transitioning to buying local, your priority is to put out the best product in order for the business to be successful. You must keep the success of the business at the forefront at all times throughout your changes.

If certification is your goal, you need to make a broad range of changes to reach 100 points. That will determine how you plan for your implementation. Ideally, you want to combine a couple of small, inexpensive changes with a major change that will save you money over the long haul. Knowing that you will be saving money down the road may allow you to look at an additional change that could increase immediate costs but absorb the hit over time. In the long run these changes will cancel each other out, from a financial standpoint; typically it will end up in your favor. From an environmental standpoint, you could double the benefits.

Repeat this process a year from now, and then a couple of years from that. The process will always need to be tweaked because we are at the very beginning of the green technology available for everyday businesses. As you set your goals, set them with an immediate game plan, a short-range plan, and a long-term plan. Using your proper planning, your fiscal benefits will be realized over time.

It is all about mind-set. Once your mind-set has changed to realize that all your actions have consequences, and those consequences are far reaching, you begin to focus on making sure you are making the right moves. I've found, in my new approach, that I catch myself wanting to make a change because it is time to reorder something and I want to get the greener product. I wish I could say I stop myself and follow my plan, but most of the time that is not the case. For really expensive reorders I manage to hold back, depending on how busy we have been. The great thing is I'm not the only one having these issues. The rest of the staff is constantly offering suggestions for ways to change and begging to implement them. The impact on staff morale really is evident. It has been refreshing to know they are behind the changes as much as I am.

Fourth tāyst

Chapter Eleven
Beeswax Candles

What's in a candle? Restaurants from casual to fancy have them on their tables burning day and night. There are so many variations of restaurant candles, from paraffin to battery to disposable to electric. Why is the flickering light so integral to the ambiance of the restaurant? Obviously, in the higher-end dining establishments, when the lights are dimmed a candle illuminates the area around the diners. It's as if you have pockets of light at each table personalizing the experience. Yet doesn't a spotlight fitted with soft lighting provide the same experience? Or does it have to have the flicker? When *tāyst* first opened we tried to minimize the table decorations and chose fresh flowers as opposed to candles. I don't remember our reasoning. Quickly after opening, we added candles to the tables, a decision based on customer feedback. People had to have their candle on the table. Unbelievably, it was a serious deterrent for their patronage. They were actually pissed. Ironically, since going green we started sourcing our flowers from a small organic farmer. As you would expect, they were unavailable in the winter, and after last winter the farmer ceased to sell them commercially. We have not had flowers since and have yet to receive even one comment.

Changing our candles was one of the initial four changes we made under the old certification system. As with most of those steps, my first thought was, *Hey, this is an easy change, let's do this one.* I proceeded to follow the same procurement strategy as I did for food. After all, it had been successful, why couldn't I also find a local producer to supply candles? There was plenty of local honey, plenty of bees. Logically, there should be someone making or willing to make beeswax candles.

Little did I know that we actually burned somewhere in the realm of 5,000 candles per year. HOLY CRAP! Think about those restaurants you see using the disposable candles knowing that they aren't likely to be recycled. In order to find a local producer we had to know what we were using. We assessed and evaluated our candle usage. It should be relatively easy for you to do the same. We tend to be regimented in some of our operations, and candle usage is one of those areas. We were lighting our candles, which were paraffin at the time, every day at four o'clock and let them burn until we closed, somewhere between 10 p.m. and midnight. At the beginning of the day we would check all the sconces and if a candle was low, it was moved to a table in order to use every millimeter— every penny counts. We had two different sizes of candles, but each fit into our candle holders. So we averaged six hours of burn time a day over five days a week. Multiply that by the amount of candles we needed—tables, bar, and sconces—and we knew exactly how many candles we used in a year. (Or, you can pull your invoices and tally what has been ordered, whichever is easier for you.)

Knowing the number of candles is not the only bit of information necessary for making this green switch. We needed to know our exact cost of the candles in order to accurately make a comparison and subsequent evaluation. With the variation in candle sizes, just using case prices wasn't enough.

PARAFFIN

Paraffin (petroleum) candles for restaurants are sold by burn time and in a variety of sizes. We used a fifteen-hour and a thirty-six-hour votive style. Now, the name is supposed to represent the amount of hours the candle will burn. But we did some extensive tests with varying sizes, burned in different environments. Not once did the burn time match the stated number of hours. In fact, on average, in each environment we were shorted 15–20% of the burning hours promised. We called the companies to voice our concern over the fact that we were paying for a certain number of hours and being shorted the total time. We received an unexpected response. We were told *we* were not burning them correctly. (Silence.) I'm sorry. We are not burning them correctly? Yes, everyone, there is actually a correct way to burn candles for maximum efficiency. That's what I get for being a cook. I definitely do not remember candle burning being a topic covered in culinary school. Once we found out the "approved" candle burning environment we noticed that it was eerily similar to what we were doing. *Huh.* Regardless, we added that to the factor for costing out our candles for the year. It basically came down to an hourly number, two cents per hour to purchase paraffin candles.

Right about the time we started researching the potential switch to beeswax candles was the first intense increase in gas prices. A price hike had just come through, bumping our cost to about twenty-five cents per hour, and you could see the next one on the horizon. At this time we weren't set on the switch to beeswax. It was actually a toss-up between switching to 100% PCW paper for menus or beeswax candles. Either one would fulfill our certification requirement for a change. We ended up doing both, but the candle change happened first.

BEESWAX

Before any of these comparisons could happen we had to find a beeswax candle. As I said, we tried to find a local source. I followed the path I had used to connect with my local farmers and went to markets looking for the bee people. I found some great honeycomb but no one who could produce the volume of candles I needed.

Next stop—the Internet. This was my first experience with how much work it was really going to take to be involved in achieving a carbon-neutral restaurant. A great number of beeswax candle companies are out there. I pulled about ten different companies off the list and started calling. Initially, I was just finding out basic prices, size options, and burn times. After going through the first great candle experiments I knew that I needed to verify the burn time claims. In this case a 15–20% difference would add up to a significant number on the bottom line. For the most part the companies were very willing to help out and send samples. The problem was nobody made beeswax candles for restaurant use. Some of the companies had variations that could work in the right votive glass—another issue we had to think about—but they were too big and didn't fit in the candle holder or they were too small and the flame was lost. Everyone was making glorious all-natural beeswax candles . . . for home use only.

Trial and Error

I was getting a lot of samples and following the same burn testing we had done previously. We had the same problems with the shortened burn time and, of course, called for the proper way to burn the candles. Wax candles don't play like paraffin ones. They have an entirely different set of nuances. Nuances such as: You should only burn them for three to four hours at a time in a draft-free environment. A draft-free zone is impossible in a restaurant setting, but the time restraint was possible. The problem with a draft is that the candle will have a tendency to heat more on one side causing it to burn unevenly and eventually cause wick issues. Any significant drafts will also blow wax onto the sides of the holders; although this seems to be a sconce problem more than a table problem, as they're closer to the air vents. Another difference is the increase in labor hours for the cleaning and replacing required as the candle burns away, as opposed to the pull and dispose method of the paraffin candles. Each glass votive must have the little bits of candle remnants scraped away each day in order to fill it with a new one. Did I mention that these containers are glass? Votives will inevitably need to be replaced.

As we broke down the cost of burn time for the beeswax candles from the varying sources, not only could we not find a candle that fit, but they were averaging ten to twelve cents an hour. By fit I mean that we had existing candle holders on the tables that we liked, and there was no need for the added expense for new ones as they already fit the décor. However, for these holders you just dropped a paraffin container into the holder. A beeswax candle needed to be in a glass votive in order to fit into these holders. So we needed a standard sized candle that would not only fit into an affordable votive but into the candle holder as well. The ten to twelve cents per hour was also at the burn time they were claiming, not what it was burning in our environment. We eventually found a company, Bluecorn Naturals, which realized the potential market of beeswax candles for restaurants. This became the first of many relationships in which we grew with a company starting to meet the demands for sustainable supplies. Even now, three years later, the market of sustainable restaurant supply is incredibly young; new technologies, systems, and equipment are being introduced with ferocity. With this particular company, the size issue was a non-issue as they were already focused on producing a restaurant votive. The major challenge was getting the cost down to a reasonable number. They started experimenting with a soy/beeswax blend that could significantly cut down the cost. By combining this new blend of candle with bulk purchases we got the price down to just around eight cents an hour. Basically, the decision came down to two cents per hour for paraffin or eight cents per hour for this beeswax blend.

The concern and reason for the debate between the paper and the candles was the dramatic increase in cost—about 400%—for the candles. This is one of the times that going green significantly affected our bottom line with no financial payback down the road. However, there was a bonus to purchasing these candles and that subsequent increase in cost. I will talk about this in greater detail later, but it was a concern we've had from the beginning: How do we deal with the skeptical customers and potential accusations of greenwashing? With all our modifications and the resulting broadcast of what we were doing, we were going to receive considerable media attention (we hoped and were right). It was inevitable that

170

people sitting at a table were going to question and ask for proof. (Maybe not directly, but there would definitely be discussions.) We believed we needed to have something tangible and in-your-face for the doubters. What better way to reinforce the signs and statements than an illuminated representation of our environmental standards? Yes, it is still a release of greenhouse gases, but we had already fought the "no candle on the table battle" and lost. So we ended up with a compromise of our ultimate purpose, but a positive selection of the best option for natural renewable fuel.

A Glowing Recommendation

It was there, on every table and in every sconce. No one could miss it. We added to the reinforcement by lighting each candle when the guests were seated. This actually served two purposes. It forced the recognition of the candle and it cut down on the amount of candles we burned by only using them on active tables. Knowing the increase in cost, we had to change the systems we had in place in order to extend the life of the candle. This step had an impact fiscally, operationally, and behaviorally.

As with all new products there were a few growing pains with the first few batches. The wicks were too high, thus increasing the speed of burn, or too low, preventing the burn altogether. The wick moved and slid to the side as the candle burned, heating the votive to a point where it would shatter. I must say that one was more than a little nerve-racking with guests sitting underneath. Eventually these growing pains worked themselves out and the candles have become a major talking point among the guests, just as we had hoped.

There were great pros to the purchase of the candles as well. Besides beeswax being a 100% natural fuel, it burns brighter, cleaner, and longer than paraffin candles. It is naturally honey-scented, a feature that is unfortunately minimized by the soy blend. It emits the same light spectrum as the sun. It releases negative ions to clean the air and invigorate the mind. Basically, it's aromatherapy. It makes people in the surrounding environment feel better. It's a really smart move being that we're a restaurant trying to make people relax and enjoy themselves.

Illuminating Experience

We had an understanding that the price would eventually go down. As the demand increased, technology could be integrated in order to make the process more cost effective. It has gone even further than that. The company split into a second company, Goodlight Natural Candles, focusing on a sustainable palm tree oil. Their journey is an excellent example of the path toward sustainable practices. As we move forward we need to evaluate the products we are using and transform them to sustainable methods. Goodlight connected with the World Wildlife Fund's newly formed Roundtable on Sustainable Palm Oil (RSPO), a certification group formed to transform the palm oil industry. The palm oil industry, at one time, had been a major reason for deforestation, erosion, and habitat loss as well as poor working conditions and unfair wages. Palm oil is one of the most used vegetable oils in the world and produces ten times more oil per acre than any other plant. It's a non-GMO tree that lives for twenty-five years, producing fruit each month.[87] It is exciting to note that the RSPO certification is changing the industry from one of

172

destruction to one of permaculture. Other companies are recognizing these needs and joining in the efforts to provide sustainable alternatives on a commercial level. We are seeing changes that not only make a difference for the environment, they are making a difference in everyone's budget. Happily, our cost after switching to this candle is now equal to that of a paraffin candle. Eventually the green way will also be the less expensive way.

Chapter Twelve
Light Bulbs

Now for the light-bulb dilemma. It's hard to believe that choosing a light bulb for the restaurant would be as hard as it has been, but eight months into my search I was still using regular floods. It's a tricky thing picking light bulbs for a restaurant. The ambiance of a restaurant is a significant factor in its success. If people don't feel comfortable with their dining experience, they will not be as inclined to return. So as we looked at switching from regular lights to energy-saving bulbs we had to keep this in mind. As always, we were hindered by the lack of funds.

The first step was highlighting the areas of the restaurant that needed to be changed. For us there were five distinct areas: outside, men's bathroom, ladies' bathroom, kitchen, and dining room. Four of the areas were a simple switch to CFLs. I'm pretty sure everyone is aware of CFL lights by this point. Even former president George W. Bush signed an order to have all government light bulbs changed to CFLs. (A CFL is a compact fluorescent light bulb that was introduced in the 1990s. You know, the squiggly bulbs.) They offer the same light output as an incandescent bulb while using much less energy—anywhere from 60–80% depending on where you look. The light is actually just a reformed fluorescent light that has been in use for more than 60 years. In order to achieve maximum lighting in a smaller area, the light bulb is coiled back around itself to provide more surface area. The average lifetime of a CFL is 10,000 hours compared to the 1,000 hours offered by incandescent bulbs. Incandescent bulbs waste 90% of their energy in generating heat. One 27-watt CFL can save 730 kilowatt hours (kWh) over its lifetime, which is enough electricity to power an average home for a month.[88] Conversely, using a CFL can prevent 2,000 pounds of CO_2 from being released into the atmosphere and restrict eight to sixteen pounds of sulphur dioxide and NO_2 emissions.[89]

CFL PROS AND CONS

The big argument against integrating CFLs is the fact that they use mercury. Yes, CFLs contain mercury, each bulb holding somewhere between 1 mg and 5 mg. This is, once again, a choice that boils down to the greenest option. If you are concerned about the mercury in the light bulb getting into the waste stream and ending up in yours or your customer's bellies via fish, it is a valid concern. However, there are a couple of facts to consider about mercury and CFLs. First, if the bulbs are recycled correctly, and almost all local governments now have a recycling station for CFLs (most hardware stores will recycle them for you as well), there will be no mercury from the bulb released into the environment. Will the occasional bulb break allowing some mercury to escape? Yes. However, in the United States, more than half the energy we use is produced by coal.[90] And since coal releases mercury as it burns, mercury is a side-effect of most of our lighting sources; however, all incandescent lights over 40 watts release approximately 75% more mercury than CFLs, so CFLs are clearly the better choice.

The savings in energy use provided by the CFLs will allow lighting fueled by more clean energy, reducing the use of coal, thereby offsetting its mercury production. A report by the

United Nations estimated that "in 2000 there were 145 metric tons of mercury added to the solid waste stream in the United States. If 200 million CFLs, each containing 5 mg of mercury were placed in the solid waste stream in one year, they would add only 1 metric ton, or less than 0.7% of the total annual mercury load in the waste stream."[91] So while the mercury argument should be taken into consideration, the benefits of the CFL with proper handling far outweigh the potential mercury contamination.

Another complaint about CFLs is that the light that is released can react poorly with some environments. The lighting industry actually has a very sophisticated Correlated Color Scale for its lights. I won't go into great detail on that; but, basically, there are four different color options: a super bright daylight, a bright light, a cool light, and a warm light. The wattages vary, but the equivalent incandescent wattage is printed on the light bulbs so it is easy to determine which you need and have an idea of lighting with similar style. For instance, a 65-watt flood will be a 15-watt CFL. We chose the 24-watt daylight CFL for outside floods. These provided us with a light that was equivalent to about a 100-watt bulb with the most power we could get.

CFLs are a great advantage not only for their energy savings, which is 60–80%, but for their durability—they last ten times longer than incandescent bulbs. We have a total of ten outside lights. They have been in for about three years. We used to replace one, if not two, lights a week. It was a running joke in the restaurant as my former partner would, very dramatically, pull out the long-handled light-bulb changer and perform the light-bulb dance both inside and outside. We kept waiting for Cirque du Soleil to drive by and offer him an act. At $5 to $6 a pop it was a pretty costly issue—somewhere between $250 and $300 a year. This, of course, is not taking into account the cost of direct kilowatt usage.

The initial output of dollars for outside CFLs was about $11 apiece. So we doubled the cost of the bulb initially, but ended up spending about 50–60% less on bulbs for just ten lights for the year. Again, this does not take into account the savings through energy conservation. So, you see, this is completely contradictory to the argument that energy-efficient lighting is way more expensive. These lights are a great example of why you definitely need to think long term when making your green decisions. So, in the three years we have had CFL bulbs in the outside light fixtures we have replaced one bulb. And that was thanks to some spring winds that loosened the bulb and caused it to fall, not because it burned out. Fortunately it fell in a flower bed and we were able to recycle it. That one-time cost was almost double, but we have saved almost $750 in replacement costs since switching to those lights.

We followed suit in the bathrooms and the kitchen with the purchase of CFLs that had the least amount of wattage with the right color—warm light for the bathroom and daylight for the kitchen. These places were the easiest to fix because they were set in their lighting schemes and didn't need a lot of lights. We also have yet to change any of them, an especially nice bonus in the kitchen, where on the hot line the lights were always going out during service. Changing lights while cooking over open flame was always fun.

FINDING THE RIGHT FIT

The dining room is where we struggled the most. Lighting is so crucial to the ambiance of any restaurant, and ours uses about sixty bulbs for the bar and the main room. When we transformed the restaurant from the previous space we were fortunate in that we had existing track lighting with bucket lights already in place, including backup buckets if and when we needed them. For a typical incandescent 65-watt dimmable flood it worked fine in our scheme and doubled as a great money saver on the front end since replacing lighting fixtures is expensive. Taking into account the fact that we only use the lights for about six to eight hours a day, and 75% of that time they are dimmed pretty significantly, we have had to replace maybe four or five light bulbs in five years. Murphy's Law, however, is the true ruler of restaurants, and as I crept closer to finding a green light that worked in the dining room, the incandescent lights started to blow almost daily.

The LED Dilemma

In researching my lighting options I had to find a bulb that had a dimmable option. This drastically limited my choices. As far as green lighting went, I had two choices: the CFL market, which had just begun producing a dimmable option, or light-emitting diodes (LEDs). The LED is considered to be the next generation of energy-efficient lighting. It is even more efficient than a CFL, lasting up to ten times longer. It doesn't have the mercury issue and produces almost no extra heat when operating. It is sturdier because it doesn't employ filaments, and, although much more expensive at the outset, will save money over time. An article on the Discovery Channel site describes them:

> Basically, LEDs are just tiny light bulbs that fit
> easily into an electrical circuit. They are

178

illuminated solely by the movement of electrons in a semiconductor material, and they last just as long as a standard transistor.[92]

I got lucky with my LED introduction. I was approached by a salesman who represented a company, Eco-story, which specialized in energy lighting. He initially brought a couple of the standard LED bulbs—one bulb was about 12 watts and the other was 4 or 5 watts. The 5-watt light is the LED wattage for a light output equivalent to that of the 65-watt incandescent. Unfortunately, their light was so specific that it caused distinctive circles to be cast along the walls and the tables, and they were not dimmable, so the brightness was overwhelming and uncontrollable. With that, I laid out the specifications of the light that the restaurant would need, and the rep went to find one that would fit. The only downside to the LED that I could see was the cost. The bulbs averaged $35 per unit, which would put us right around $2,200 to outfit the room. As with all of the energy-efficient equipment, I once again had to weigh the cost against the return. We were looking at a fourteen-month time frame for the return on the investment and then savings for each year to follow. Amazingly, the lifespan of LEDs is around 50,000 hours, so they could outlive the restaurant.

My next round of lights for testing took about six weeks. You might be wondering why it took six weeks to get a new bulb for testing. (I wondered the same thing.) We ended up in the same situation as the beeswax candles. The light bulbs existed, but they were in the early stages of development, and each time I sent back my representative with a tweak to the light, he had to go back to the design company for the development of a completely new light bulb. By this time, green lighting was really starting to gain traction, and I had an opportunity to participate in a webinar covering the history, structure, and benefits of LED lights. The webinar was beneficial in that it described the problems and solutions other companies had encountered, particularly with LED selection and installation. Of course, the main difference between these companies and mine was budget. One restaurant chain in particular, Chipotle, had the business most similar to mine, but their usage was not quite the same—bright versus my need for dim. Their answer to the distinctive lighting pattern, the bright circles on the walls I mentioned earlier, was to add more lights. There was absolutely no way I could afford to add more buckets and consequently more LEDs to fix the problem. I had to continue my search for a solution.

Seven or eight months later we were on attempt number five or six. Each time, we tried to warm the light as well as widen the beam spread, to about 80% coverage underneath the bucket, to get as close to replicating the incandescent flood as possible. The structure of the LED is a very bright solid light. It produces a straightforward beam, thus its initial use in clocks, flashlights, Christmas lights, etc. In order to fix this and transform these lights into functional daily lighting, the designers were starting to add diffusers to the top of the beam, in order to spread the light out, as well as reconfigure the construction of the light by using a number of smaller lights within one bulb. Color blending was also being developed to try to soften the light being emitted. All these advancements are still in the early stages as this type of lighting moves into the mainstream.

Part of my concern was to find a bulb that would provide the lowest wattage possible to maximize my energy conservation. As I stated earlier, we had about sixty buckets to replace. Each bucket held a 65-watt incandescent. The lights are on about eight hours a day, five days a week, fifty-two weeks a year, give or take a few days. That means each bulb pulls about 135,200 watts of electricity per year. Multiply that times sixty and you're up to just over 8 million watts per year on just the bulbs in the dining room. Eight million watts is 8,000 kWh, which puts out an average of about 1.3 pounds of CO_2 per kWh, or 10,400 pounds of carbon into the atmosphere.[93] It was a priority in my greening efforts to significantly reduce, if not eliminate, this output. There is a secondary factor of energy conservation that is provided by using LEDs—the decrease in heat emitted. Incandescent bulbs produce heat as they operate, about 85 British Thermal Units (Btus) per hour compared to the 30 Btus per hour by CFLs and 3.4 Btus per hour used by LEDs. The extra heat from incandescent lights collectively raise the temperature of the room, causing the air conditioner to work a little more and a little longer to keep the room cool. LEDs put off almost no ambient heat eliminating the secondary energy impacts.

I could have given up and gone to a dimmable CFL. It is a great choice, regardless of the mercury debate. But after months I had to ask myself: *Is one choice more sustainable than the other?* Maybe, but if my budget only allowed me to switch a few to LEDs compared to being able to change all of them to the CFLs, what is the best way to go? They do conserve energy, about 31,000 watts per year rather than the 135,000 for incandescent lights. CFLs were definitely my fallback, but at that time, I had not yet given up hope that I could find an LED that would work. As with everything we've done in greening the restaurant, we were not willing to just give in and take the easy road. I really wanted LEDs in the dining room and if there was a viable solution that made good business sense, I was determined to find it.

I listed a number of the benefits of the LED previously, but its most appealing attribute is that it is the best energy-conserving bulb out there. One of the coolest aspects of the bulb is the fact that there is a 70% lateral decrease in wattage with a dimmable LED. That means that with a 12-watt dimmable LED we would be able to limit our usage to about 4–5 watts of electricity, basically around 8,500 watts per bulb per year. To look at a direct comparison: 8 million watts from incandescent to .5 million from LED usage. Plus, it comes with a three-year warranty. When an LED fails, it is typically part of the hardware in the light that goes, not the bulb itself. The hours provided by the manufacturer represent the light burning at its full potential for the determined hours. At the end of that life cycle the light will not blow or burn out, but it will dim from its initial output. Basically it will perform at a lesser rate. LEDs would be the last lights we ever purchased for the dining room.

Near Misses

By the end of our experimentation, we finally found, or I guess designed and had manufactured for us, a light that had the color we needed, a beam spread that covered the area like floods and dimmed in an acceptable manner. After the amount of time we put in, I was ecstatic not only to find a bulb, but to finally start conserving the energy in that area of the restaurant. Then I got the price, $60 a bulb—$3,600 to outfit the dining room. I just didn't have the funds. I had wasted all that time developing a functional LED only to find I couldn't buy it.

Devastation. I couldn't believe that the initial quote I was given was half of the actual cost. I tried some negotiations with the company to get the price down, but it just wasn't going to happen. They were working on some new technology that would be ready in a few months, maybe, that should work in our scheme for our price range. I tried to look elsewhere. I checked with a few other companies and received some samples, but we were back to square one. There wasn't a bulb being produced that could fit into an existing lighting scheme like ours. I tried Eco-story one more time to see if any progress had been made and found out they had gone in another direction completely.

Settling

I had to accept the fact that I was going to have to get dimmable CFLs. Again, not a bad choice at all, but I know at some point in the near future there will be an LED that fits our needs in our price range. This is the downside to being passionate about shifting to and maintaining green operations. For those of us who recognize the need to find green options, things will be more expensive. But, as with food, the more of us who participate, combined with advancement in technologies, the sooner these options will become mainstream and more affordable. The light bulb saga is a great example of the process for a lot of our changes. Assess, evaluate, and decide what we want to do. Find possible sources, find out they don't actually fit our needs (either functionally or fiscally), hopefully convince them to make one for us or find someone who will make one for us, and get it to fit in our price range. Pretty simple, really.

Just as I had come to accept the CFL move, I attended a Green Business Summit—a three-day conference and business expo. What should I find, but an LED supplier? And a new one at that! It was a new variety of LEDs from what I had found so far. Instead of one, three, or six lights within a housing it was a grid of 20 to 100 very small lights. Same color options, same possibility of increasing the beam spread. They would be a better fit because they eliminated the distinctiveness of the individual lights within the housing. It was the answer. The color and the spread were not as difficult to fix as the distinctive beam. This had to be the bulb. And it was . . . to the tune of $100 a bulb. Back to CFLs. I didn't see them at the summit the next year.

Finally, Success!

A few months after the summit and eight or nine months of research, trial, and error, the search for bulbs was over. After resigning myself to the dimmable CFL, we started a cost analysis for a dimmable r30 CFL before purchasing so we could get the best deal. During this process we came across a company that had just released a dimmable 5-watt CFL. After all this time and effort trying to make an LED work for the added savings in wattage (which had been our focus), we found a CFL that equaled the wattage savings. The best part: it was $8.49 a bulb. After a quick call for samples to make sure it provided enough of the right color light and fit within our ambience, we were sold. Final cost for dining room plus a few extra bulbs was $636.75, as opposed to somewhere in the thousands.

There are some negative aspects of the CFLs that have been exposed recently. Complaints about the length of time the bulbs actually last are popping up, some manufacturers' bulbs in certain lighting fixtures will blink or make noise or the light doesn't come on instantly. The bulb life issue seems to be related to the number of times the light is turned off and on. A fixture that is used repeatedly will tend to burn out quicker than a light consistently used. However, the lights on motion sensors in our bathrooms have not yet burned out and are turned on and off numerous times in an evening. As far as the noise/blinking issues, it's about trial and error. If one light blinks, you can return it and get a different brand.

I will receive the same savings, financially, as I would've with an LED and at a much faster return. The downside is that the lifespan will be much less than the LED—according to the manufacturer it's 25,000 hours, compared to 50,000 hours for the LEDs, but most CFLs are rated at 10,000 hours, so we will see how long they last. We had one other unintended consequence. When we experimented with the samples in one area, the lighting seemed more than adequate. Once the whole room was lit with 5-watt bulbs we no longer needed the dimmers and it was quite dark. We could work around it, but that might not be the case for other restaurants out there. Take the time to find a light that works within your scheme, but make the effort to make the switch. You'll be glad you did.

Chapter Thirteen
Take-Out

To-go containers may be the easiest and the hardest green change you can make. It is an easy fix because in the last few years the amount of choices has increased tenfold, but again, it is a hard fix because there is no definitive right choice. Are you as tired of that issue as I am? Why would to-go containers be such a big deal? Well, in 1969 the United States produced 270,000 tons of disposable plates and cups. In 1997 that number jumped to 1.8 million tons. In 1994, 39 billion pieces of cutlery, 113 billion cups, and 29 billion plates were produced. Less than 1% of these products were recycled.[94] If you combine that with the new information on how often we eat in our cars—approximately one out of every five meals—or that the school systems are serving their meals on Styrofoam plates with sporks, the amount of take-out disposable containers we are using will only continue to increase.[95]

The first required step to achieve certification from the GRA, in either format, was to remove all Styrofoam from the premises. I think most people know the evil of Styrofoam is that it doesn't biodegrade. As it enters the landfill at alarming rates, typically with food residue, it breaks into smaller particles. Animals are drawn to these particles through the aroma of the food residue and ingest them, clogging their throats and digestive tracts.[96] Unfortunately, there are other issues that really make it an even greater environmental foe. First, it is made from petroleum, a nonrenewable resource. According to the American Chemistry Council website, Styrofoam constitutes less than 1% by weight of landfills in the country; yet one of the benefits of Styrofoam is that it is 90% air. The fact that it is mostly air and made with petroleum is why it is cheap. This, of course, along with its weight, is why it is widely used, not just in the food industry, but throughout industry in general. More can be shipped for less in a lighter package. Second, the actual production of Styrofoam itself causes air pollution and health hazards for those involved. "Acute health effects are generally irritation of the skin, eyes, upper respiratory tract, and gastrointestinal system. Chronic exposure affects the central nervous system; symptoms such as depression, headache, fatigue, weakness, as well as minor effects on kidney function and blood can occur."[97] While in landfills not only will it not break down, it will crumble to fine pieces eventually being eaten by wildlife, which makes its way back into our food supply. If incinerated, it releases toxic material into the air and into your food when microwaved.[98]

TAKING IT TO-GO

Recent years have brought a boom to the recycled and biodegradable product lines. When we first tried to move to an environmentally friendly option we went through our local Sysco distributor. Following is a recurring story of the problem of supply and demand, particularly with Sysco. They brought in a product for us to use, after we used all of, what I assume were their samples, it was gone. They would no longer bring it in because there wasn't a market and it was too expensive. We had to find another source, which we did, and since then even more sources have emerged. We have actually circled all the way back to Sysco with their new eco-friendly product line, which they introduced with great fanfare, about a year after they told me they were done with it: The wave of the future

187

and what your customers want, they said. I chuckled as I sat through the presentation. Yet, we need companies like Sysco to get on the train. If I have to go through the same experience for every product for them to move towards the right food and supply, so be it. In the end, they carried it.

Currently, there is an incredible amount of choices all claiming and offering an environmental benefit of some sort. Even the Styrofoam websites tout its environmental benefits, expectedly I suppose. In reality, as far as restaurants are concerned, there are two choices within the environmental lines: bioplastics, primarily poly-lactic acid plastic (PLA), and a vegetable starch variety of molded fibers. Both are made from renewable resources and both are continuing to make strides in product variation, quality, and cost. The technology is moving very quickly in this area, however, and new products are being introduced regularly.

PLA Plastic

PLA plastic is made by transforming a starch, typically cornstarch, into a resin by converting the dextrose to an industrial lactic acid. The resin is then manufactured into a plastic product. Many starches such as wheat and beets can be used to derive the lactide needed to blend the long-chain polymers which turn into plastic. In the United States, corn is king and that's the type of starch we generally use. PLA plastic is the next most affordable container after Styrofoam and only a little more expensive than the recyclable petro plastic varieties. The benefits of using this material are the elimination of toxic substances, a 65% decrease in energy usage during production, and a 68% reduction in greenhouse gas emissions.[99] When properly handled it can be composted, incinerated, or recycled. When it comes to functionality, it rivals the petro plastics or petroleum-based plastic containers in its offerings of shapes and sizes. However, it does have some drawbacks.

Opponents of the recent push for bioplastic production, primarily the PLA plastic, claim that it is being praised too quickly. It is following the path of bioethanol, a path receiving high praise before there was a true understanding of its environmental effects. In reality, it can only be composted in commercial composting facilities, of which there are only 113 nationwide. Additionally, even in the commercial composting system the PLA plastic returns to lactic acid, making the pile acidic, requiring more oxygen for the microbes.[100] When it makes its way to landfills it acts no differently than regular polyethylene terephthalate (PET) or other petro plastics, another issue that comes up during the recycling process. The PLA plastic is hard to distinguish from petro plastic. Essentially, when PLA plastic gets into the recycle stream of petro plastic that stream becomes contaminated and everything goes to the landfill. That means we rely on the observance of people to make the right decision to dispose of the product properly, if they even know that they need to do so.

From a restaurant perspective, the major drawback is the melting point, which is around 114 degrees. You cannot put a high temperature sauce in it or you will be cleaning up a mess. I know from experience. That being said, technology is moving quickly and starch-based resins are beginning to be manufactured to deal with this heat issue. In my view, the major drawback to PLA plastic, especially in the United States, is the use of monoculture industrial GMO corn in its production. Here we are attempting to manufacture an environmentally friendly product from a renewable resource when, in actuality, the base for the product has significant negative environmental effects. Supposedly the bioplastic industry is moving toward more low-fertilizer, low-pesticide products like switch grass in its production. In fact, as early as this year a bioplastic produced from switch grass is supposed to hit the market. The polymer is grown in the leaves and the leftover residue can be used for biofuel. [101]

Bagasse

The other option in the earth-friendly take-away container world is a wide variety of fiber mold products made from vegetable starches called *bagasse*. These products are being manufactured using a number of sources, mainly leaves, wheat, sugarcane, limestone, and grass. I am really just scratching the surface in the types of molded products available because we don't do that much to-go business, but to me they seem to be the greenest option. We are using a sugarcane by-product made from the pulp left over after the initial processing. The containers are heat proof, freeze proof, and will compost in your home compost bin.[102] They are also the most expensive variety on the market right now. We eat the cost because it's a minimal percentage of expenses with our limited usage, and, like the beeswax candles, it's another bit of tangible evidence to satisfy the skeptical guests.

WEIGHING THE OPTIONS

Here we enter one of the major debates in the green world, or at least in our green world: What is the best option? Let's look at the options, starting with the cheapest, and the worst.

Styrofoam is gone. The negatives far outweigh the positives. Actually, the only positive thing I can say about Styrofoam is cost. The next option is recyclable petro plastic. It is relatively inexpensive, and it can be recycled, but it is made with a nonrenewable source. Better than Styrofoam, yes, but since the price is tied to the cost of oil, it can only go up. The real benefit of petro plastic is the functionality. It holds hot and cold, and there is a size or shape for every restaurant in the country. Bioplastics are next with only a marginal increase in cost over petro plastic, if that is even recognizable now.

There is a drastic decrease in functionality with the inability to hold hot product, though that concern is probably going to be resolved soon. There is the fact that it is a monoculture corn product. Again, from a cook's perspective, monoculture corn is worse than petro plastic. Can we really call it a renewable resource? We know that at some point the amount of chemicals used will have destroyed the soil enough to reverse the yield per acre. Some, like Julian Cribb, author of *The Coming Famine*, at the recent International Foodservice Sustainability Symposium (IFSS), say it's already happened with yields per acre around the world ceasing to improve if not starting to recede. As the industry potentially switches to a renewable resource, it may become the best option, but for now, I feel it's on par with recyclable petro plastic. The last option, and the one we chose, is the bagasse—vegetable starch mold. Ours is a sugarcane by-product, heat resistant and compostable. It is more expensive and for the few to-go orders we do produce, we put it into 100% PCW bags, which cost about 75 cents each, making it even more expensive. If I had a restaurant that did more to-go business, I think my choice would be more difficult.

Yet again, there is no clear cut answer on the best product. Even the sugarcane has some downside. The containers don't close perfectly and there aren't that many size or shape options to fit your needs. When someone needs a doggie bag it costs us about 50 cents to give them a container to put it in, and if we put it in a bag, that goes up to $1.25. That cost adds up at the end of the year. Also, if the sugarcane isn't organic, it is probably burned in the fields before harvesting, which does not necessarily leave a small carbon footprint. However, it is a by-product, so it is being made from a product that used to be waste and was burned at the end of the day. This use of what was once a waste product, to me, makes it the best choice.

Some other things to think about while you are making your decision: As mentioned before, you have to rely on the guests to recycle it or compost it. Most people won't save their containers until they find the correct way to dispose of them. If the trash is right in front of them that's where it goes. Knowing that and knowing that recycling is probably the only likely option if it doesn't go straight into the trash, it is even more important to choose the option with the least impact as it goes in a landfill. The answer is definitely restaurant specific. In a more casual restaurant that might be more focused on to-go orders, I would have a hard time deciding between petro plastic and PLA plastic. I have to say, the corn use really bugs me. Ideally, I would lean toward a bioplastic made from switch grass. I would also seriously contemplate a small dollar add-on for the containers so I could use the vegetable fiber brands. In normal times that would probably be fine, but in recession times like these any added cost should be considered very carefully.

Chapter Fourteen
Waste and Recycling

Inextricably attached at the hip are waste and recycling—one necessitated by the overload of the other. We waste lots and lots and lots of products in all aspects of our society, and the restaurant industry is—though I hope to change it—a perfect example. It is estimated that one restaurant can produce 50,000 pounds of garbage per year.[103] A ton is 2,240 pounds, which means that one restaurant potentially produces just over 22 tons of waste each year. According to the National Restaurant Association (NRA), there are currently about 960,000 restaurants in the United States. We'll round up to 1 million for easy numbers. At that number the restaurant industry is producing 22 million tons of waste per year. I actually feel the number is quite higher. One report from the city of Los Angeles states that one restaurant actually produces 50 tons of organic waste per year (organic waste is 76% of a restaurant's waste output).[104] That potentially places the output of a single restaurant at about 62 tons per year and the overall restaurant output at 62 million tons. Even at the NRA's 22 million tons, the industry is responsible for almost 10% of the waste stream.

According to the EPA, the total waste stream in 2009 was 243 million tons, with 82 million tons being recycled. As you can imagine, the recycling percentage has significantly increased since 1990. Unfortunately, the amount of waste produced per person has also increased. In 1960 the average waste produced per person per day was 2.68 pounds; in 2009 it was up to 4.34 pounds. The rate of recycling in 1960 was 6.4%

and rose to 33.8% in 2009.[105] Of this Municipal Waste Stream (MWS), or garbage, "33.8 percent is recovered and recycled or composted, 11.9 percent is burned at combustion facilities, and the remaining 54.3 percent is disposed of in landfills."[106] That's still quite a large amount going to the landfill. Just so everyone is on the same page, when the MWS goes to the landfill it is not so it can decompose and disintegrate, it's so it can be covered up and forgotten about. Covered waste in a landfill is restricted from the two key ingredients to decomposition, water and oxygen.[107] But the main problem with using landfills is that you will eventually run out of land. However, we do seem to be heading in the right direction for waste management, except where food waste is concerned.

Food waste is defined by the EPA as "any food substance, raw or cooked, which is discarded, or intended or required to be discarded. Food wastes are the organic residues generated by the handling, storage, sale, preparation, cooking, and serving of foods." Food waste in America in 2009 totaled 33 million tons with only 3% diverted from the landfill.[108] It is the second largest segment of the MWS at 14.1%, just ahead of yard trimmings at 13.7%, plastics at 12.8%, and behind paper at 28.2%. Factor recycling into the MWS and food becomes the clear-cut winner for solid waste disposal at 33.44 million tons, with plastic following at 27.71 and paper falling back all the way to third at 25.93 tons.[109]

WASTE MIS-MANAGEMENT

I am throwing a lot of statistics at you in order to frame the waste stream so we can understand the impact food has on a sustainable future. The trends are easy enough to see. Waste is increasing, but so is recycling. At the current pace, recycling could potentially eclipse waste in the future. The exception to this is food waste. The individual stream of the MWS increasing at the highest rate is food waste. *Science Daily* recently reported that "US per capita food waste has progressively increased by about 50% since 1974 reaching more than 1,400 Calories per person per day or 150 trillion calories per year."[110] This equals enough food to feed 2 billion people a year, yet many are starving. Americans are wasting roughly 40%, although some reports say 50%, of the food we produce.

Stop and think about this assessment and what has happened over the last thirty-plus years. Fast food has increased, restaurant portions have increased, food has become cheaper, waistlines have become bigger, health has worsened, and resources have begun to show signs of stress. Basically, it's all the issues we have been discussing. At the IFSS lecture Julian Cribb made an excellent point relating how the cheapness of our food has resulted in a lack of respect for what we eat. How else can we throw away almost half of our purchases? Try this: Take all the money out of your wallet, purse, or pockets and throw half of it away. Would you do that? No. Or, how about this: Go to the store and buy two chairs, throw one of them away. No? It's mindboggling when we think about it. Add to this the political unrest in many parts of the world that is being driven partly by high food prices, or the response in this country as beef and dairy prices are expected to rise 5–10% over the next year. Arguments against a local or regional food system are so often centered on price, but factor in how much food we waste. If we can eliminate that in tandem with buying the right food, the prices would immediately come in line.

Who's at fault? How did we get to this lack of respect? A big part of it is our need to feel we are getting the most for our money—the supersize meals, the buy two get three free, the discounts, the deals. Regardless of why, this food waste issue is a direct result of failing to understand where our food comes from combined with our distorted notion that we have to have platters of food if we are going to get our money's worth. Quantity over quality is an unfortunate aspect of the American way right now. To think that our health issues are not related, as previously discussed, is naïve.

There are other negative repercussions to the exceptional amount of food waste produced, an issue not solely based in North America, by the way. A report by the U.N. Food and Agriculture Organization (FAO) stated that the world food waste number is a whopping 1.3 billion tons a year or a third of the food produced in the world each year. This, of course, has a ripple effect. "Food loss and waste also amount to a major squandering of resources, including water, land, energy, labor and capital and needlessly produce greenhouse gas emissions, contributing to global warming and climate change."[111] American food waste alone is responsible for 300 million barrels of oil and one quarter of freshwater use annually.[112]

There is a difference between waste and loss, however. The FAO report specifies that food loss occurs at the production, harvest, and storage stages of food production and is typically an issue in developing countries. Small farmers do not have the resources, funds, infrastructure, or technology to properly handle the harvest. Whereas in developed countries the food waste occurs at the retail and post-retail stages, in which case food might be tossed because it isn't perfect to look at, though it is perfectly edible. Another cause for waste is when too much was purchased. Amazingly in both developed and developing countries the food wasted is the same, about 670 and 630 million tons, respectively.[113]

Reduce

Circle back to waste in restaurants and the first thing to think about is that almost everything in the restaurant industry is recyclable. The GRA says this amounts to 95%, while the Zero Waste Zone project by Elemental Impact in Atlanta says that it's only possible for restaurants to recycle 85%. The Zero Waste Zone project is an initiative by the city of Atlanta to tackle the issues we are discussing in this chapter and to eliminate or rather to alter the current waste stream to one that is completely recycled. Several times in this chapter I have listed multiple statistics. I have done so in order to show how early in the game we are. It is difficult to compile exact facts partly because of the variety of establishments within the industry. Numbers for fast food, casual, and fine dining are going to be quite different. This means there is incredible expense in funding a study for exact restaurant waste statistics. Regardless, each number—95% and 85%—is stunning, and both show that, as an industry, we have the capability of making a significant environmental impact through waste management.

Recycle

Recycling was one of the first changes we made in greening the restaurant. Within your "garbage" you have different streams of waste: organic or food, paper, plastic of numerous varieties, metal, and glass. Every city has its own regulations on recycling. Some cities, such as San Francisco, are very proactive and offer full recycling, including composting. Others, like mine, offer no commercial recycling pickup whatsoever and limited residential recycling. We do have locations or drop-off sites in which recycling occurs, but hauling a restaurant's recycling to a certain location a number of times a week is unrealistic. I am not saying that transitioning to recycling has to be mindless and easy in order to work, but it also can't be so difficult that it becomes prohibitive.

My first step toward developing a recycling program was to call the local government, where I promptly found that I was out of luck. Next step: cold calls through the phone book and Google searches. There were a few scattered services but nothing that actually offered a solution. At that time we were sharing a dumpster with our landlord, using the waste behemoth, Waste Management.

Reuse

We were already recycling cardboard, but they had yet to offer any other recycling services. I say "yet to offer" because Waste Management is now going after the recycling market hard. According to one of their vice presidents I met at a conference recently, they are starting to treat their existing landfills as gold mines by excavating them for plastics that can be turned into crude oil, among other things. They are experimenting with a number of operations to capture the discharge of gases produced by the landfills and transferring that energy back into the grid. They are starting to build compost facilities and more.

Similar to the moves that Walmart is making (even if money might be the only driving force), if recycling gets the industry as a whole moving, I see no problem with it as a start. As far as Waste Management picking up our recycling, it wasn't an option. Our certification would have been okay with just cardboard recycling because that was all that was offered in our city. This was just four years ago, and Nashville, though a fairly major city, barely had any recycling going on whatsoever. I was shocked. That wasn't enough for us. Then I got another break and found a company that was starting to offer recycling to commercial businesses.

As usual, it was a new company that saw the market and wanted to capitalize not only on the newfound desire of businesses, but also people's desire to do the right thing. People want to recycle. They want to keep trash from going to the landfill. The best part of this company, EarthSavers, is that they would take glass as well. As I said, they were just starting out so I feel we kind of grew together. The recycling pickup was a multi-stream can for paper, metal, and plastic and a single stream can for glass. It seems that nationwide, glass pickup is the hardest to coordinate. A number of factors contribute to this. The first being that special trucks and equipment are required deal with the glass. Glass breaks. The little pieces have a tendency to find their way into the machinery of the trucks, equipment, etc. The mechanism breaks, repairs are expensive, and it becomes cost prohibitive quickly. Cost is the real deterrent, however, to glass recycling. Besides the repair costs that can be attributed to the broken glass, it costs more to make recycled glass than it does to make new glass, and there is no shortage of sand—the biggest ingredient in glass—out there. Add the cost of the recycling process to the glass-making process compared to that of sand sourcing and there is little incentive for businesses to add this to their services. Everyone knows that recycling costs money right? If the process isn't fiscally sustainable, then it will not be a solution to the waste system for very long. All facets of the operation need to be funded and a market for the material needs to exist.

Sorting It All Out

Separation is a major part of all recycling and one of the major costs. Remember, in order for an item to actually be recycled, it must be made into a new product. Just because it was thrown into the recycling bin does not mean that it's recycled. Collection is not recycling. As I said, EarthSavers collected everything mixed together; they would then sort it before delivering it to the manufacturers who would turn it into the new raw material. As a smaller company, they sorted manually at the time. Technology is moving fast though, and for larger recycling operations there are now materials recovery facilities (MRF) that are incorporating food production line systems into waste recycling. They are eliminating the sorting costs attributed to labor by using a mechanized line with magnets, air vents, and rollers to separate the waste into the right streams.

One big problem with recycling is contamination. Materials with food residue, wet paper, little tops, all of these things disrupt the stream, causing product meant for recycling to be diverted back to the landfill. I will admit that we had more than one angry call regarding contaminated recycle streams. However, ours was more related to the improper disposal of things. The soiled paper towels, which are actually compostable, plastic wrap and aluminum foil, and plastic or latex gloves were all materials that continually found their way into the recycle bin. Pre-recycling, we used five trash cans in the kitchen, one in the server area, and two behind the bar. All of these cans would end up between half-full and full nightly, get bagged, and tossed into the dumpster. We removed the cans from behind the bar and replaced them with one for glass and one for mixed recycle plus a small compost bin. In the kitchen we removed all the "trash" cans and now have one recycle bin, one compost bin, and one trash can, which, even on the busiest of nights, we will fill maybe halfway. We went from eight trash bags in the dumpster each night to less than half of one. Using numbers, we went from eight 60-gallon trash cans, or 480 gallons of trash, to less than 40 gallons, DAILY. We have since tried to minimize the product that can't be recycled by using an already recycled product, such as aluminum foil. If we have to send something to the landfill, at least it is not a new product. The reason aluminum foil cannot be recycled is that foil with food scrap tends to burn up during the recycle process.

There are a lot of numbers to be found that support recycling, but rather than regurgitate a bunch of statistics on the environmental benefits, I thought it would be better to offer statistics regarding the waste stream as a whole. We all know that recycling is a better way to go. Even my six-year-old understands the importance of recycling. In a restaurant, it is pretty easy to get to the place that you have almost no waste. The monetary benefits are simple: You will pay less for waste disposal through decreased usage if you recycle. You might also have to pay for recycle pickup, depending on where you live, but the cost should end up in your favor. EarthSavers is getting ready to incorporate a trash bag pickup along with their recycling pickup. That would save me about $2,500 per year in my dumpster cost (and I only pay half of the total fees).

I mentioned compost, but I haven't really discussed its incorporation into the restaurant. Compost is the one area where every city should focus their efforts. I am actually in discussion with Earth Savers to develop a citywide composting program. We'll see what happens with that. As we saw with the increasing food waste each year, it is the one area in which we, as a country, are currently making no progress. I was fortunate in that I struck a deal with one of my farmers that allows me to close the circle for part of my operation. Karen Overton with Wedge Oak Farm—a new farmer getting back to the family land—came to me with a proposal to take my compost. I was just starting to use her for chickens, eggs, and pork (all of which are exceptional), and she was interested in my organic waste. So she takes my compost, makes awesome dirt, dirt makes good bugs, good bugs make fat chickens, fat chickens taste great, food scrap from preparation goes back into compost, repeat—a closed circle. The only downside to this cycle is that it works for us because we are small. As we eventually incorporate more restaurants into the mix we will need an improved system for compost development and distribution along with a way to pay for it all. Although I seriously doubt we'd have difficulty selling a good amount of killer organic compost to local gardeners.

The importance of composting in a restaurant is, obviously, the decreased amount of waste that would otherwise end up in a landfill. Organic waste is the worst ingredient in the landfill because, as it breaks down, it produces methane, which, as we know, is twenty-one times worse than CO_2 as a greenhouse gas. Landfills overall are responsible for 20% of methane emissions, most of which are produced by organic waste.[114] By diverting this stream completely we can produce a vibrant soil that is drought resistant and reduces the need for irrigation, fertilizers, and pesticides. The development of compost facilities could be costly on the front end; but, they could have a huge impact on so many aspects of a sustainable future, particularly climate change and food production. This doesn't even include the food added back into the system from eliminating the needlessly wasted product. Just focusing on this as a solution to the worldwide food crises might be the simplest attack of all. You could argue this solution against both sides of agriculture—that it is easier than re-regionalizing a farm/food system or developing a GMO strain that has no negative repercussions.

Reduction of waste, proper recycling, and composting are the trifecta of multi-purpose solutions. The many layers of positive change that can come out of these simple practices will have lasting effects on the sustainability of our food sourcing production and food supply.

Main tāyst

Chapter Fifteen
Initiating the Change

Now what? The decision is made, the assessment is done, and the evaluation is over. You have a solid understanding of the pictures and the reasons for moving forward. You've decided which steps will be your focus. You have decided whether or not to be certified. You are at the point where you are ready to start putting the changes into action. Hopefully, throughout this book, you've noticed the underlying similarity in the formula we used for all of our changes. It was a formula that has been, and will continue to be, successful for each step we attack. I believe this formula will evolve as our industry moves forward, as technology provides more choices for those who want green options for their operations. I also believe that what are now green options will, in fact, become standard as our industry progresses. However, as we are still in the early stages of the game, the formula we used in our product search has been a proven success and one you can easily adopt, and it's always better to be the proponent of the change instead of the follower. I am going reiterate how we changed our food purchases as an example of the green transition.

Obviously, we have discussed the food aspect quite a lot because, to me, that is the key to a sustainable future. I'd like to ask you to take a moment to think about the historical implications of fluctuations in the food supply. Consider food in relation to major events, social changes, and cultural movements throughout human existence. As I mentioned earlier there is an overwhelming connection to the constant battles over the control of the food supply, such as the one happening in America right now, between the real food movement and the current food system structure. Throughout history, civilizations have been so focused on protecting their food supply that wars were fought over the control of fertile land. It was a driving force in the development of the world today. As noted food historian Reay Tannahill said, "For 50,000 years and more, humanity's quest for food has helped to shape the development of society. It has profoundly influenced population growth and urban expansion, dictated economic and political theory, expanded the horizons of commerce, inspired wars of dominion and precipitated the discovery of new worlds."[115] It is quite ironic, really, that one of the key elements in molding our civilization has been all but eliminated from the thoughts of most of the population. If you no longer think about how our food comes to us—beyond the grocery shelves—how can you know if the supply is in a healthy state? Even more, how can you know if it is not?

LAYING THE FOUNDATION

Food was the very first change we made; granted, it was a few years before we consciously made the connection between the food system and the health of the environment. But, in hindsight, it was my very first green business move. For everyone out there already focusing on local purchases, you, too, have already started on the path to greening your business. For those looking to start local product integration, your first step is finding farmers. Where do you start? Use the Internet. Most states have an agricultural database of all their farmers listed within the state Department of Agriculture. You can't sell food without a USDA permit and must register to do so, thus the comprehensive listing. Typically, contact information is also available and you can start cold calling. More and more, I am finding that even some of the smallest farmers are set up with websites or at least an e-mail address. If you are not getting enough headway with your Internet searches, then magazines such as Nashville's *Local Table* are popping up in various cities with the purpose of connecting the consumer to the farmer. We are fortunate that ours provides a list of almost all the farmers in our area. If that list isn't available, there should at least be a list of farmers' markets in the area with dates and times of operation, and farmers' markets are increasing exponentially. Since 1994 the number of markets has increased from 1,755 to 6,132 in 2010. In the last six years alone the number of markets has almost doubled.[116]

BUILDING THE SUPPORTS

As I stated in Chapter Three, "Local and Sustainable," make the time and go to the markets, meet the farmers, buy their product. This farmer search will eventually lead you to other farmers providing different products or maybe more of a specific product you need. I relate the farmers at markets to independent restaurants. On one hand, we are competitors, on the other hand, we all want each other to succeed. So, at least in Nashville, we band together for greater strength. As a group we fight the advertising and purchasing power of the corporate chains like the small farmers at the market are fighting the huge power of industrial agriculture. The relationship that develops out of consistently buying from local farmers will result in a reversal of roles, and new farmers will begin to seek you out. Once you reach this point, you have successfully made your mark in the local agricultural community and are on a solid path to becoming primarily locally sourced. That is the basic formula for building your green food infrastructure. Apply the same approach to finding items such as the aerators or light bulbs. Start with a wide search and whittle it down until you have a couple of reliable options. The only difference is that the face-to-face component of food sourcing is critical to success, where you can do much of your operational product sourcing online.

As you begin to make changes, one of the most important things to consider is the natural shift in your mind-set. The importance of a solid assessment and subsequent plan development really solidifies once you begin to make the alterations. These will not only happen in your business, they will seep into everything you do. I chose to weave the stories of my experience into the data to explain the rationale for a green restaurant because they are representative of how the process will affect not just the way you operate, but the philosophy you embrace for how you live your life. I didn't know that much about being green before I started on this journey. It was a learning experience every step of the way. I have learned more while writing this book than I ever thought I wanted to know about the environment, and I still feel as though my understanding is very superficial.

We are restaurant folk, and it is ridiculous to think that with the few hours left in the day we can attempt to assimilate the many layers of information on all the environmental issues. No one is going to start on this path with all the answers, if all the answers even exist. If there were solid, already determined solutions, I would be willing to bet that a lot more restaurants would already be green. It's the way most revolutions work and how the green movement is overtaking the country right now. As more information is reaching more than just the diehard tree-huggers, people are acting on that information. The truth about the lack of limitless resources and "the unlimited growth in a finite world"[117] is being heard, and businesses are jumping on the bandwagon. That, to me, is the most obvious clue. When every business is trying to find a way to showcase their green efforts, it represents the true desires of the consumer. It's an infectious virus spreading through the country.

OPENING DOORS

Viral is a good way to describe what happens. You get the bug, and it begins to take over. Before you know it, everything you do has the potential to be greener. For the most part, people want to take care of the earth—they want to sustain what gives them life. It's an innate urge to prolong human existence. It starts with one change, such as putting aerators on your faucets. Soon you realize that the aerators are good, but you can also fix your toilets. Next you cut out the running-water thaw technique to conserve water. The change of these habits or operations leads to a desire to replace your A/C unit because it represents almost 25% of the water you use. Maybe you can't really afford to do that, so you try to cut down on the use of the unit with window film or other methods. You get the picture. Our biggest problem, and frustration, has been postponing desired changes because of financial restrictions.

We get psyched about the opportunity for putting in this sensor or replacing that piece of equipment and forget we don't have the funds necessary to make that step. It is continually disappointing to know that there is so much more you can do to reduce your carbon footprint, but there isn't more room in the budget to make it happen. That is why developing your plan is so important. Look at your finances, figure out where your funds will come from, and what the return on your changes will be, and then decide on a timeline for your changes. Stick to your plan and timeline no matter how badly you want to keep changing. Learn from my mistakes so you don't face the same pitfalls in deviating from your plan, experiencing a surprise drop in business, and find yourself choking through a month with a kink in your cash flow.

Another valuable component to remember as you initiate your vision is to make sure you let people know what you are doing. Find ways to tell people you are taking steps to benefit the environment. You can reach an entirely new demographic of customers who will support you and your efforts. The benefit of tapping this demographic is that they are very loyal and very connected. Like foodies, greenies talk among themselves and to their friends about supporting restaurants that use local food or are being socially conscious. The downside to this demographic is that they are also the people who tend to go to the market and cook at home a lot. Eating at home means they are not in your seats.

So what do you do to get the word out? This can present a tricky situation depending on your restaurant setting. There is a fine line between educating the customer by providing information they should know and bombarding them with data that doesn't enhance their dining experience— where the food comes from, for example. In all this local food source/use discussion we mentioned time and time again that it's about building relationships with your farmers. Well, people eating in your restaurant also want that relationship. They want to know where their food is coming from, but that can be accomplished simply by listing the farms on your menu.

Now, if we tried to list every single one of our farmers on the menu (i.e., Farmer Dave's parsley root), we would end up with a menu that is twelve pages long. We would need to sell advertising in order to support the associated printing costs. And that presented a dilemma we had to address. How do we communicate to people the amount of local food we are buying without printing it on the menu? Enter: "the chalkboard." I went to the parent-teacher store and bought a big chalkboard and placed it on a stand my wife found at an antique store. Total cost was $30. On the top I wrote "Nashville's First Certified Green Restaurant," and then I listed all the farmers whose product we used that day. It has been the best piece of marketing I have ever done. I think it may have been photographed more than my food. The most important aspect of the chalkboard is not the fact that it lists our farmers—although, to me, they are the key to my success. Actually, they are the key to everyone's success because farmers are actually the people who feed the world. My farmers deserve all of the recognition I can give them. But the big deal about the chalkboard is that it gets people talking, and the more they talk, the bigger the conversation becomes and the more people learn.

Restaurants are more fortunate than other businesses in that they have direct, face-to-face contact with every single customer. We have an unbelievable opportunity with that direct contact that not all businesses can mimic. As more and more businesses make the switch to green practices and, in so doing, wish to separate themselves from the pack, they must simultaneously avoid claims of greenwashing. It is important to maintain this contact with your customers in a manner in which it elicits a positive response—to balancing your communication with them so you aren't in their face, but still get the word out about your efforts. It's a difficult task, requiring creative solutions. These solutions will vary with the style of restaurant. A casual sandwich shop can be much more open and direct than a fine-dining establishment that requires subtlety and finesse.

Because of where it's positioned, every single customer who walks through the door of our restaurant walks by the chalkboard. Inevitably, for those new customers or those who do not know that we are green, it hopefully sparks questions to the server. Yes, some see the list but don't read it, which creates an opportunity for the server to bring that selling point into the menu discussion, which can become a bigger conversation. We take the subtle approach. During their introduction, servers will mention the farmers on the chalkboard. With an understated mention of the chalkboard and the green certification we open the door for the customer to choose whether or not they would like to hear about our practices. It's less intrusive, but a great way to spark interest in what we do and why we do it.

You will find your biggest challenges are in changing your food. It is by far the hardest aspect of greening your restaurant, particularly if the local food infrastructure in your community is still in its early stages of development. This is not to say the other changes are easy, but they mostly involve doing research, listing the options, and selecting those that best fit your operation. Food sourcing is more complicated and requires more legwork and relationship building, but trust me, it will be some of the most enjoyable and rewarding work you do in this process.

The key to remember as you begin the changes is to stick to your plan. You spent a lot of time and effort assessing and evaluating your options. You made a plan that takes into account your current and future budgets. Once you are on the path to making a difference, every little bit that you do is important. Slow and steady wins the race.

Chapter Sixteen
Results and Impacts

I think I have made it clear that this book has taken me a very long time to finish. I've heard it can take around two years to write your first book. Counting a year of planning (and procrastinating from the fear of how difficult it might be), it will be a little over three years since this project began. It has been just shy of two years since I first wrote this chapter. What I find exceptionally interesting is that as I started to revise this chapter, which focused on what had happened post–green certification and the impacts this move had made, there was very little I had to add or revise even in the wake of the ongoing recession. The results are the same and the impacts have not only remained in place, but have actually intensified.

What has happened in the last three years has been nothing short of miraculous. Perhaps it can be said that the right way won't be denied, that it will eventually force itself into existence. The local food movement and the green movement have evolved into a legitimate force in politics, business, and economics. There are still decisive battles going on in each of those forums over the right course for the environment. I don't know if we will ever resolve that debate in a democratic state, even more so in one so dependent on the use of nonrenewable resources; unless, of course, some of the scientific projections come to pass. If we begin seeing increased ocean levels, continued rise of climate temperatures, crop yield reductions or loss, food safety issues, greater health issues, or unaffordable transportation costs, we might focus less on arguing and more on acting. Let's hope that these projections don't have to become reality in order for us as a society to change our path.

EMBRACING THE CHANGE

As we settled into the flow of being green at *tāyst*, we quickly realized there is no such thing as routine. In our pre-green life, the days only varied with business, at menu change time, or the occasional wine dinner, but the general routine was relatively the same. We were constantly attempting new creations and had days that were a total cluster f@#$. But, for the most part, those issues were becoming small pieces of the puzzle that is our restaurant day. With this new system of sourcing, of constantly looking for farmers, plus the new practices for being green, the work toward a greener restaurant has not stopped. (I'll let you know if it does.) After service one night, I was sitting with a few members of my staff and we began to debate what the response would be from our impending announcement. Would there be backlash? Would people think it's nothing but a PR stunt? I considered these and some other pessimistic thoughts that ran through my head. It was that same last-second bit of anxiety I feel as a cook before putting a dish out there. Will they like it? Is it great? My bartender/GM Adrien looked up and sternly made the comment, "How often is what's 'good' for you, actually what's good for you?" There was an amazing truth to that comment.

When we started this process it quickly became about more than just turning the business green. It may have started out that way, but it definitely evolved into much more. It was a learning process for me and my staff about the state of our environment, and, more importantly, where we are heading and what we can do about it. I now realize the wealth of knowledge I have been fortunate to gather while going through (and even after) the certification process. I am constantly trying to learn more about all of the issues relevant to my goals. Obviously, these issues are important and complex enough that universities now feel it is necessary to offer advanced degrees in sustainability with a food system focus. In the beginning, however, I didn't have the knowledge. I went forward based on a gut feeling that it was the right move. There were still a few doubts. By stopping, stepping back, and taking a holistic view of the system I knew I made the right move. That comment from A.D., my bartender/front-of-house manager, regarding what is good for you hit it right on the nose. As the web of connections unraveled I knew that, regardless of the response, we were doing the right thing. Really, what bad things could people say? I am aware that there are the anti-climate change activists and individuals who don't believe we are actually going to run out of fossil fuels. There are those who are naysayers, who are going to swear we did this for PR and nothing else. We hoped those people would be a small percentage. I am a chef; so even though approval from others is paramount, I still have a tough skin and can handle criticism (most of the time). My staff and I had worked so hard toward these goals that I didn't want them to be for naught. I wanted to be sure that the response was loud and positive.

When we finally sent the e-mail announcing that we had been certified "Green" by the GRA—the first in Nashville—and one of about sixty or seventy nationwide at the time, it garnered some attention. We received write-ups in magazines and papers, local TV features, and other press. They were all very positive articles relaying my evolution from the passion for locally sourced food, to its connection to the environment, and the need to apply those beliefs throughout the entire restaurant, reinforcing the chef-driven nature of the business. We got enough exposure that we ended up landing a gig catering a Martha Stewart wedding that was produced for the Style Network. We have now launched a green catering company called Local Kitchen Catering as a result of the interest stirred by the special. We did a spot with CNN when they were in town covering the green surge happening in Nashville. The response from my regulars and my new customers was overwhelming. Even after realizing there really weren't any negative responses to what we were doing, I was still taken aback by the positive comments and interest from the community. Not only was it obvious that we had done the right thing, it was obvious it was what the people wanted.

BRINGING OTHERS ON BOARD

The reaction was so positive I discovered the tremendous ability that restaurants have to make noise in their communities. Whether it was the advent of the Food Network and celebrity chefs or the "foodie" population, the fact is, when a restaurant does something different it is always big news. Chefs and restaurants have the community's ear. Maybe it is a fallback to the times when the restaurant/pub was the hub of the community. When it was the hearth of the community. Regardless, it is a great thing to be in an industry that can reach so many people. The positive press we were receiving was affecting more than just my business. The best result was that the farmers were reaping the benefits as well. Each article that was released listed not only where I was getting my product, but how to go about getting some on your own.

I started to field calls from other restaurant folk who wanted to sit down and find out what it would take to start their restaurants on the path to being green. Some were owners, some were chefs, and some were just employees. It didn't really matter who they were, it was the fact that they were asking, that they were interested. It wasn't always for a full-on greening, some people just wanted some advice on to-go containers or a local dairy. But that didn't really matter.

Before I knew it I was becoming involved in a lot of places besides my restaurant. I never planned on becoming an activist. In fact, I made it clear on numerous occasions that I was not trying to be a lightning rod for the issues at hand. Initially, I just wanted to show people it could be done and it could be done successfully. I wasn't interested in talking (I know that is a shock to those who know me), just doing the walking.

JOINING FORCES

There was something about the viral nature of the changes I made. They were initially a by-product of the search for knowledge, but that search included the discovery of organizations seeking the same solutions to the issues we've been discussing. They might be related to health care, food source, or poverty. Maybe they are with environmental organizations. There are a lot of groups both locally and nationally focusing on issues with the food system.

Each national group had a food forward focus. The Slow-Food movement focuses on the preservation of food traditions. The Chef's Collaborative seeks the establishment of a sustainable food system. On a local level I became very active in a group called the Food Security Partners. This group really hit home with me as it is a centralized organization with which other groups could partner. It serves the purpose of bringing together different entities interested in fighting for a just food system. Their mission is simple and straightforward: "Joining together to create and sustain a secure and healthy food system for Middle Tennessee, from production to consumption." It really is very similar to Chef's Collaborative except it focuses on a specific region and goes beyond just sustainable food.

By joining these organizations I have been able to make contacts nationwide with individuals with the same focus. This has not only reassured me that we are headed in the right direction, but, after a recent conference, I've also discovered we are pretty far ahead of the game. I have attended conferences to debate food-related issues and learn some "best practices," as well as participating in the discussion to determine what exactly is sustainability. I joined a number of these groups for educational purposes, as well as giving myself an excuse for business trips; but with the Food Security Partners (FSP), there was another purpose.

In the beginning, my work with this group stemmed from my abhorrence for the state of the food in the school system. One of the main emphases of the FSP, which is now called the Community Food Advocates, along with addressing food deserts (areas in which access to healthy food is difficult, if not impossible), was their "Healthy Kids" campaign. Programs and initiatives like this are spreading throughout our country, led by groundbreaking chefs Alice Waters and Ann Cooper, seeking to return local healthy food to the school systems. Maybe it's because I have children who were just starting in the public school system, but I quickly realized the added benefits of fixing the food situation in schools.

CHANGING THE COMMUNITY

In Nashville there are 78,000 children in the public school system. Of those children, almost 70% are on the free and reduced lunch program, and half of those students get almost 50% of their nutrition from school, and an unlucky few receive 100% of their "nutrition" through the school system. This school issue is not a new discussion. Everyone—books, TV shows, Oprah, Jamie Oliver—is talking about it, and for every negative story there are success stories and there is a solution. The government has recently updated the regulations for school food for the first time in years. You might read this and think that it does not pertain to the purpose of this book. I bring it up for a couple reasons, the most pressing being that teaching kids about real food at an early age will give them a better opportunity to develop a palate that craves healthy food instead of processed junk.

Another reason directly correlates with the theory proposed in this book that chefs can save the world. We know that any successful alteration of the food system will have to allow variances from region to region. Every region has a school system that, for the most part, is a perfect picture of that region's demographics. By successfully integrating a sustainable food system within a school district we will have developed a blueprint that can be expanded to the greater region. In order to procure the amount of food necessary for supplying the schools, a local food infrastructure that is affordable and accessible must be developed. A chef is typically involved in the menu development and procurement of food service in the school system. He or she has direct control over what is purchased. The challenge, of course, is meeting government regulations in order to receive the federal financial reimbursements—each meal must meet certain nutritional requirements in order to be considered a reimbursable offering by the USDA.

Unfortunately, even within the existing sustainable food world some question the necessity of the fighting the school food battle as well, of including it in the push for a sustainable food system. If you are truly working toward a sustainable food system I see no way not to be involved. For more information on this issue and the efforts in your area, check out Chef Ann Cooper on the Internet at http://chefann.com and her Lunch Box Project at http://www.thelunchbox.org to see some of the things she is doing. It is obvious to me that the answer for many of our health, food, and environmental issues lies in the foundation we are laying for our children in the food we are feeding them, the land we are leaving them, and the future we are mapping for them.

The allotted amount of money available to school systems to feed two-thirds of their kids is less than a dollar a day for food. The federal reimbursements are about $2.76 and include labor and supplies. Just this year they were increased by a whopping 6 cents, the first such increase in reimbursement in years. I suppose the politicians just don't understand that if we can teach this generation of kids the importance of food grown with environmentally friendly practices and how to eat properly, we could reverse the unhealthy trends.

We've made some progress in the four years we have been fighting for school food changes in Nashville. It took three years to get to the table for a discussion, and a year later we are seeing the potential for transformation. One thing that has stood out more than any other during this battle is the power of our youth. There are many people donating countless hours and energy to this cause, including a number of very bright students. When they speak, people listen. They have the power to get their peers behind the difference we want to make. They are proof that our current food system is inadequate and that people recognize the need for change. They are your future customers. They have done their part, we just need to deliver.

REACHING THE RIGHT AUDIENCE

To me, the answer is the children. One of the main reasons I really bought into the green beliefs was the anticipation of what our children are facing. Is it not every generation's responsibility to leave the world a better place for their children? Again referring to the tobacco fight, the children were the ones who made that battle successful. As we educated them on the negative effects of smoking, they went home and harassed their parents about quitting. I understand that we are all having serious budget issues in every public school system in the country, but it's time to reevaluate the systems preventing us from moving forward. Studies have shown that a child who is fed healthy food at school will go home and request healthy food.

That child's desire still leaves us with the dilemma not only of the family's access to get healthy food, but their ability to afford it. Complications presented by food deserts and the deficiencies of school food are as intertwined as all the other issues we face. We have not yet come up with the perfect answers to help our communities. As with everything, each community must find a solution that will work for their unique obstacles and requirements.

One of the impacts of our sustainable business philosophy includes community involvement. As one restaurant, I was able to develop an infrastructure that makes my small neighborhood restaurant work. But one of the reasons I operate the way I do is to advance the food system as a whole in order for it to be easier to do my job. However, a secondary concern is creating a world where my grandchildren will be able to have real food. I have been fortunate to take it a step further through my involvement in Nashville's first Food Policy Council. Food Policy Councils are beginning to form all over the country with the purpose of advising the "Powers-That-Be" on issues surrounding the food system in the hopes of passing, enacting, or altering planning policy that includes a sustainable food system and accessible food for everyone. We are still finding our legs, but to be a part of such an endeavor is a great experience and a great honor. I have the opportunity to improve the food system within a region and develop a sustainable food supply. We have the great privilege in Nashville of really making a difference that has a national reach. Nashville, to me, is the greatest example of Middle America. Systems which we put in place here as a mid-sized major city are the types of systems that could potentially be implemented around the country.

Overall, the results of going green have been overwhelmingly positive, and the impacts are greater than I ever expected. Running your own restaurant is a dream come true for everyone in the beginning, but the relentless difficulty of the work can weigh on you no matter how passionate you may be. The love of food can even be diminished by the all-consuming work. For a short period, turning my restaurant green doubled the amount of work we had to do to continue to operate. This was, in part, because I have a very small staff, but also because we were just starting out and it was harder to find solutions. Yet, instead of becoming discouraging, it was invigorating. It led me to be more involved in my community because I believe in the system we have created at the restaurant. I also believe these solutions should be easier to find and afford, because this is a system we should use as a country. Green is good.

Chapter Seventeen
Defining Sustainability

Sadly, defining the term *sustainability* that is so central to our discussion is a monumental undertaking that really has no answer; yet it is still the one thing people want to know. What is sustainability and what makes a sustainable restaurant? Some say it's all about the food, others say the operations are what matters, and others still, like me, believe a holistic view is the key. The restaurant industry is one of the biggest players in the current industrial food system, creating a significant percentage of the U.S. contribution to climate change. Again, animal husbandry alone is responsible for one-fifth of the carbon emissions, and agriculture overall produces more than one-third of our country's carbon output. Add to that the fact that the restaurant industry is the biggest user of energy in the retail sector, emitting a major amount of carbon, and this equates to a significant amount of damage to the climate. However, unlike the energy industry or the agricultural industry, it isn't controlled by a small few. In the restaurant industry there are no large conglomerates deciding how things will be done or where the money will be spent. "Big Ag" doesn't force us to buy their food, neither does Sysco, Performance Food Group (PFG), or any of the other processed-food providers. Even the largest conglomerate of chain restaurants is a small piece of the pie.

So as we push for these operational alterations while moving toward a greener industry we have to convince more than just a board of directors or a few CEOs. We need to be able to provide solid information that will entice people to *want* to change. As we have discussed, the industry margins are so small that the willingness to modify a business model that is making money is difficult to find. We need to be able to define what a sustainable restaurant entails, demonstrate the process required to get there, and prove that it can be equally as profitable (or more so) as one that is environmentally unsustainable. It's time to decide exactly what a sustainable restaurant will look like, even though we know an urban restaurant will take a different shape than a rural one. A sustainable restaurant in Tennessee will function differently than one in New York. That fact, among others, is what makes this so difficult.

Much like the food system in general, the interplay of parts that make up the restaurant industry (or on a larger scale, the hospitality industry), is such a tangled web that the task of establishing a blueprint for sustainability might be insurmountable. Fortunately, I am a firm believer that everything is possible, so let's clarify the goal. Obviously, with enough hard work and money anything can be done, so there is potential for a sustainable restaurant industry. And, it looks good on paper. However, the reality is, putting it into practice is easier said than done.

Even with money, the players involved have to *want* to do the extra work. If they already have establishments, they have to be willing to adjust their existing operations in order to become green. This is much easier for a small restaurant than a chain of thirty. The labor pool must be educated enough to be able to utilize a local/regional food system that is different from the heat-and-serve products to which they might be accustomed. That same food system must exist and needs to be able to provide for the region completely and competitively. Consumers need to understand why this is important and be willing to accept the limitations, such as the lack of availability of a tomato in December. Farmers must return to a permaculture form of farming in which they are not using artificial agents on the farm. We have to require transparent systems to ensure proper food sourcing and safety. Companies should start providing products that supply the industry with affordable green options. Alternative energy has to become more accessible in order to supply the large need by restaurants that conversely need to decrease their own energy usage. This is just a small list of the various components that must fall into place in order to build an infrastructure of sustainability for restaurants. Basically, we need willing participants across the board, accessible product with variety, and validity of sourcing in our food purchases.

DEFINING TERMS

Let's put together a workable definition of *sustainability*, just so we're on the same page. Sustainability is, in actuality, a very simple idea:.To exist in the present, in a manner in which the world is unharmed by your presence and can continue to thrive in the future. Straightforward and simple, right? Unfortunately, the word and the idea has been overused in discussions and integrated into so many situations that its meaning has become convoluted. Are we talking economically sustainable, or politically, environmentally, or socially? Or, do we need to establish a context in order to shape the discussion? Yes, currently, without context, the definition of sustainability is too far reaching and vague to properly convey its meaning. In its simplest terms, the definition regards life on earth. That may sound philosophical and just too hippie-ish, but that is the only way the simple definition of sustainability can be used within its original meaning. We live in a manner that does not damage the earth and simultaneously ensures that it is functional for the future. Once sustainability is focused on a particular facet of this issue, the context alters the meaning of the word. It becomes more complex. Luckily, smarter people than I have already looked at the complex idea of sustainability in an attempt to demystify it.

A couple of models have been used to conceptualize sustainability: the intersecting circle model, or the Venn diagram, and the three-legged stool. In a Venn diagram, one circle is economics, one circle is environmental or ecological, and one circle is social. The area in which all three circles intersect is sustainability.[118] The other popular model is that of the three-legged stool. Each leg represents the same association as the circles in the Venn diagram and the seat is sustainability. The models afford the ability to assimilate the definition or the idea into the needed context. For instance, organic farming is economically viable for the farmers, environmentally sound for the earth, but is yet to be affordable for everyone.

Understanding the Model

Currently, industrial farming is not sustainable because it fails to meet all three criteria. Industrial agriculture is economically viable (although I'd say that is debatable), socially viable, but fails significantly from an ecological standpoint. You could also argue against its economic viability and even its social viability if we introduce the health implications and the treatment of workers into the evaluation. In fact, anti-industrial agriculture activists could argue rather convincingly that industrial agriculture is exactly the opposite of a sustainable system, failing on all three counts.

Try to incorporate this model into the restaurant industry to get an idea of a sustainable restaurant. Does it work? Is it different for each individual restaurant? Is the complexity of the restaurant operation too much for the idea of sustainability to fit? Are there even answers to these questions? Simplified: A restaurant is sustainable if it's economically viable (meaning it's making money), it's ecologically sound (meaning it's leaving the earth a better place), and it's socially viable (meaning it's accessible and affordable for everyone and pays fair wages to its employees).

Well, in the restaurant context I don't know if that model works. Economically speaking, it is pretty basic—either the restaurant is making money or isn't. From a social standpoint, the difficulty increases significantly. While I don't feel my restaurant is expensive by any means, many people see it as one for special occasions only. Many more may not be able to afford it whatsoever. As with organic farming, it's only accessible to a small part of the population. By the model of sustainability, my restaurant fails. However, in the overall attempt to define sustainability, for restaurants, I have a potential fix for this dilemma.

Socially Sustainable

Within the leg of social sustainability, restaurants are judged on a sliding scale. Our country, or the world for that matter, wants variety. With restaurants there will always be the need and the desire for different types of establishments at all levels—from a meat-and-three to über-fine dining, from $5 per person to $500 per person. We have to define

229

sustainability for restaurants with this understanding, otherwise we will never be able to outline a context in which a viable sustainable restaurant exists. Whatever definition we develop, it has to work in the current reality of the world as well as the one to come. We can't have all restaurants be the same, nor would we want that. The wages for employees in the industrial-fed restaurants, both at the establishments themselves as well as the farms involved in harvesting and processing food, are the other portion of the sustainability model's social leg. They need to receive fair wages in order to live. Those wages will be different from one part of the country to the next. Now the formula for social sustainability extends beyond the restaurant itself.

I think Gary Hirshberg put it best when he said that when it comes to greening your business it is a much bigger deal than just looking at the operations of your business. You have to look at each and every aspect, from the growth or manufacturing of the product, to the waste that the process produces, to the origin of their raw materials, to the supply line from point A to B to C to your door, and so on. Even the smallest business touches many people along the way.

Using that principle, the key to becoming sustainable seems to be decreasing the amount of layers between the raw product and your customers' plates. I'll give you an example. Will Harris, my grass-fed beef mentor has a farm in Georgia called White Oak Pastures. I have been fortunate to sample his beef but do not use it because it's all the way down in southern Georgia and I have a *local* grass-fed beef source. Will has a pamphlet that shows the layers of the beef system from the farm to the plate. His grass-fed system goes from the farm to the distributor, in his case Halperns' for restaurants and Whole Foods Market for the public, and then to the customer. One delivery from the farm to the market, then it is picked up by the customer. Industrial beef, on the other hand, goes from the cow/calf farm to auction, then to the stocker operation, and back to auction. From that auction it goes to the feedlot, to the slaughter plant, and from there it goes to the processing plant, on to the meat distributor, next to the grocer/foodservice operator, and, *finally*, to the customer.[119] Nine stops on the way to the plate.

Purely looking at carbon emissions (and no other environmental factors), this is obviously unsustainable. However, let's look at distribution using the sustainability model. Economically, even with the amount of work and travel involved, industrial beef has been cheaper. We know that this is partly because of subsidies providing cheap grain (grown in an ecologically detrimental manner), to fatten the cattle faster, thereby getting them to the market quicker. It is also because of the use of antibiotics, which allows for more head per square foot of the feedlot. There's no need to go back through these beef-raising issues. Suffice it to say that White Oak Pastures has started a box-beef program, just like industrial beef, in order to widen their reach and provide for the demand. Unfortunately, too many chefs and cooks no longer know how to break down beef, or any animals for that matter.

Also, it's not just that chefs have lost the knowledge, it's that the industry has streamlined itself, removing the time and equipment from the everyday kitchen to allow for significant animal fabrication. So, a box-beef program is a necessary program as we move toward the future. As the price of fuel skyrocketed—specifically over the last few months, but even as it has roller-coastered in the last few years—Will's grass-fed box program, besides being the better steak, is now cheaper than the industrial product. And since that industrial model is based on a nonrenewable resource it is only a matter of time before this enigma is consistent across the board with farms other than White Oak Pastures. If you have the time, check out Will's setup; it's a shining example of what can happen when you think outside the box. His formula shows the possibilities of a regionalized food system. It also demonstrates the successful blend of the current desires of the existing food system with a new sustainable production system. One has to ask, regarding industrial beef, does the economic leg of the sustainable model then fail because this beef is falsely cheap? Or because it will not be economically viable in the future as oil prices rise indefinitely? We do not even need to look at the other two legs. We know the answer. But the example shows one way to get closer to sustainability: cut out the middlemen and remove the layers of food production.

Environmentally Sustainable

Going back to the environmental leg of sustainability within a restaurant . . . it's easy right? Buy local and organic and you're sustainable. Going on the example we just mentioned, this should be even truer. If only it were that easy. Nothing about going green within the food system is black and white, as I have stated many times throughout this book. Before we even get into food, let's give a quick nod to the other functions of the restaurant that have ecological consequences and may or may not be sustainable, depending on how you operate. How about paper goods and disposables? The relatively simple answer is: use recycled 100% PCW products and or bagasse disposables. Consider chemicals. Purchase green chemicals, which are now being produced with more variety and effectiveness (a key requirement) or make your own using

232

products such as baking soda, vinegar, glycerin, lemon juice, and water.

Then there is water conservation. This is where we get into tricky territory because you can't operate a restaurant without water. Can you actually reach a sustainable level, or achieve total sustainability? Perhaps, but in order to effectively determine the level of sustainability for water use in a restaurant there should first be an acceptable form of measure in place. In this case I think there are two possibilities: first, a certain amount of CCF usage based on the size of the building, the number of seats, and the hours of operation. The difficulty, of course, is determining what that number will be. Second, it could be based on a percentage of reduction from a previously established CCF usage. A truly sustainable restaurant would be water neutral and that is unrealistic. But we do have enough information to determine a scale to evaluate acceptable water limits. The potential options provide choices for the establishment of a sustainable measure for restaurants.

Now let's look at energy. Actually, energy does not present the same difficulties as water. The easy answer is to switch to 100% clean or green energy. Even with using only a portion of green energy, it is quite possible to be carbon positive by offsetting the remaining carbon output. Currently, the likelihood of being able to afford enough solar or wind power to fully supply a restaurant's energy needs is fiscally unattainable for the majority of the industry. However, as technology evolves we will have more options than just wind or solar. Currently, you can purchase green power from the grid—the regular energy structure—although that adds a premium to your energy bill and could start to affect the economic leg. There is a new product that converts waste oil to energy that can be integrated into the operations. Or it is possible to purchase a converter that collects excess heat from coolers and A/C units and converts it into energy. Of course, all these options have expenses associated with them, and they are not yet affordable enough to put into play on a large scale. But I think the best answer is similar to that for water. Determine an energy measure formula for kilowatts used compared to the size, number of seats, and hours of operation for a restaurant. To achieve sustainability, decrease the percentage of energy used by a certain amount based on what was previously used, or do not exceed a certain number of kilowatts per hour (kWh). Neutrality of energy and water may not be realized for the near future, but perhaps those options just mentioned can get us closer to a viable answer. Maybe it's not black and white, but at this point I'll even take dark gray.

Waste is one area in which we absolutely can establish a black-and-white line. Besides latex gloves, plastic wrap, and foil with food residue, everything you can conceivably use in restaurant operations is either compostable or recyclable. A creative restaurant could get by without using foil or plastic wrap. Some say a restaurant can recycle only 90% of its waste, but I think "true zero" waste is possible.

Of course, then there is the elephant in the room: food and beverages. So often beverages are left out of the sustainable food discussion, and I would say they account for 25% of sales at most places. At *tāyst*, it's around 30%. That gives us four areas to focus on: drinks, produce, land protein, and fish. We will look at them collectively for the most part. We have already focused on the pros and cons of the options in these areas and there is plenty of information readily available to delve even deeper. You can guess by now that the complexity of each of these discussions is too great to firmly label one way as sustainable or not. But the sustainable model is effective when looking at businesses in their specific context to determine whether they are reasonably sustainable. We can use that model to look at these four areas as well, and hopefully come up with an answer that at least approximates success.

When we look at purchasing food and beverages, obviously we try to get the most sustainable product we can. The problem we still have is, what *is* that exactly? The honest answer, or at least the most ideal answer, I think, would be food grown on or right next to your restaurant, watered by rain, in soil improved by your own compost, cultivated in a completely organic fashion, and rotated to leave the soil better than it was when you started. I am not a scientist, so I am not sure if that is the absolute best answer, but it seems a pretty carbon-free solution with no negative impacts (except maybe loss of parking). Is that a realistic scenario? Unless you are Dan Barber at Blue Hill at Stone Barns or someone else with a strategically placed accessible farm restaurant, probably not. So what is the next best thing?

When we talk about the food system, do we automatically include beverages? Is that an understood part of the equation? Definitely when disposables and recycling are discussed it should come into play. When fair trade is discussed, coffee is the first product that comes to mind. The anti–high-fructose corn syrup issues bring up a number of drinks with this ingredient, but the first to the guillotine is definitely soda. The sustainable solutions are relatively simple on this front: Use bottles (re)made out of the right materials. Use the right organic products in your drinks. Stay away from the highly processed products. Then there is barley, hops, and grapes . . . all of these now have products that fit into the sustainable future.

In the beginning of this move toward sustainability, the American organic options were either not of good quality or not at an affordable price. That has all changed. Products of good value and quality are pouring into the market—organic, biodynamic, recycled glass wine bottles, solar powered wineries, etc. On top of that, the Europeans are beginning to market their environmentally friendly bottles as well. Even though it didn't require any changes, except for the label, for the most part they have always farmed their wine correctly. The one inescapable downside is that all these products must be shipped. I would love to say that I have an answer for that, but I can't. Shipping is a necessary part of the food system.

For years, the airline industry has been getting the worst rap, but recent studies are calling out the shipping actual ships—industry as well. The carbon emissions for "over-the-water" shipping are estimated at 5% of global carbon emissions, or 600–800 million tons of CO_2.[120] The airline industry contributes about 3% of total emissions worldwide.[121] Carbon emission is not the only environmental damage done by transportation, but that goes into another discussion entirely. Arguments can be made for the elimination of shipping, or at least unnecessary or excessive shipping, to all restaurants who want to be sustainable. But there is no way to remove it completely from the system. In fact, if we really want to be effective in altering the food system, we will need the efficiencies of scale that a regional distribution system can provide. As with water and energy, perhaps the answer lies in a graduated system in which the sustainability of the product shipped is taken into account as the measurement is performed.

Taking this shipping discussion across the whole food system, let's consider fish in particular. Many people like to eat fish, but a very large portion of those people do not live near the water. The impact that sourcing a sustainable product can have, compared to an industrial product, far outweighs the impact of the difference in shipping. This is that idea of traveling sustainability I covered earlier. It sounds ridiculous and crazy and critics will have a lot to say, but in the current climate, it is an idea that can exist. It is an idea that works. It definitely brings us back to the sliding scale of sustainability. At any rate, a fish caught via sustainable methods—methods that don't hurt the environment in which it was caught or risk the loss of fish for the future—which I will receive a fair price for, is sustainable, even though I have it shipped via next-day air. The carbon battle is happening everywhere, and the shipping industries, whether they be planes, trains, trucks, automobiles, or boats, are looking for greener ways to transport. They know that global trade will continue, if not increase, in the years to come and public outcry, regulations, or just a belief in doing the right thing will require a shift toward greener methods. For now, however, shipping is a part of the system; while I will minimize my use of it to the best of my ability, it is still a necessity for my business and most of the restaurant industry.

Before I move on, I do want to make it clear that I don't believe it is impossible to operate with little or no shipping. It is very possible, and hopefully one day we can get back to a system in which that is the norm. This attempt at defining sustainability for restaurants means looking at the industry as a whole, throughout the country. And we, as an industry, must give people what they want or we will not meet that economical component of the sustainable model. People want fish. People want wine. Providing that allows us to fulfill two of the three legs of that sustainability stool.

FINDING SUSTAINABILITY

I still have not answered the overall question of how do we determine the ecological leg of food? I've internally debated many ways to develop a rubric for evaluating the sustainability of food sourcing for restaurants. The three-legged stool model for the purchases of the restaurant seems to be the best approach. But the first issues you will face are the layers of hidden factors involved in the purchases. Now within those purchases it may be a simple evaluation of sustainability, but combining them in order to figure out your restaurant's sustainable level makes the task infinitely harder. That's the complication we face in the local system, the need for many farmers and enough variety in those farmers to ensure enough products. Inherently, that is also the key to fixing our food system—reclaiming farming from the conglomerate few and giving it back to the diversified many.

It also forces the realization that a clear and concise definition of a sustainable restaurant might not exist. In fact, I don't believe it does. So far, no one, to my knowledge, has really tried to hammer out an example of a sustainable restaurant because, as we have seen, the complexity of this undertaking makes it too overwhelming. However, I think we just need to look at it in a different way. I am even more positive about this after listening to Julian Cribb at the IFSS suggest a similar idea. Sustainability for restaurants should be determined on a graded scale. I've mentioned that sliding scale a few times regarding the assessment of sustainability in general. As the GRA did with the greening of restaurants,

238

allotting point totals to certain aspects of the operation, we need to assess a percentage grade to restaurants if we want to be able to rein in the varying ways to evaluate and qualify a sustainable restaurant.

My goal is to have a restaurant with no carbon footprint. However difficult it may be, I know it is a possibility. It is important to understand that even if a restaurant achieves that state, it may not be 100% sustainable, failing economically for instance. The only way to quantify these components is to develop some formulas that take into account all of the factors involved, and, I mean *all* of the factors —waste, chemicals, travel, emissions, labor, methods, profit, sourcing, etc. These formulas will not need to be adjusted for certain restaurants, but they will automatically adjust to the style of the restaurant that is being measured. The results of the formulas will compose a grade that reflects the level of sustainability for the participating establishment. The GRA point scale is a good start as it tries to level the playing field for determining the green level of a restaurant, but it needs to be more in depth in order to tackle sustainability.

Black-and-white answers? Yes, for some parts, but definitely dark gray for the rest. Until we find a method that can fairly and reasonably consider everything that is in play, the idea of sustainability for restaurants will be determined by the beliefs of the people doing the work. How significantly they want to improve the food system and their facility's mark on the earth will be the main components used to determine sustainability. Are you more worried about the use of chemicals and antibiotics, what is happening in the ocean, or climate change? Is local more important than certified organic, or vice versa? For now, it's up to us to forge the sustainable path.

239

Perhaps we should have begun by establishing the difference between "green" and "sustainable," but maybe it's an even better place to close the discussion. For a restaurant, there may or may not be an exact answer, but hopefully we can craft a model that provides a basic understanding. A "green" restaurant, or a restaurant that is going "green," is one that has made, or is starting to make, changes to its style of business that reduce overall harm to the environment through conscientious purchases, energy and water conservation, and waste management. It is a restaurant that has begun decreasing its overall carbon footprint. A restaurant can be green without being sustainable, in its strict definition, but a sustainable restaurant will always be green—a significant distinction when we talk about the importance of greening restaurants. It's like when we were in culinary school and the instructors continually reiterated a quote from, I think, Ferdnand Point: "Perfection is unattainable, but it is the drive for perfection that determines greatness." Maybe sustainability follows suit. Sustainability is perfection. It is that place we strive to be. Greening is the process, the drive toward perfection, and it is where we can all realize greatness. The ultimate greening of the restaurant is what will make that restaurant truly sustainable.

Chapter Eighteen
What the "F" is a Foodie?

"Foodie" is the most prevalent self-descriptor in the world of food to emerge in the last thirty years. The term originated in 1982 via either Paul Levy or Gael Greene, but has been broadly owned by Paul Levy. Paul actually co-authored the first book I could find regarding foodie-ism in 1984: *The Official Foodie Handbook*. A Google search for the word "foodie" yields 16,500,000 results. There are 1,420,000 blogs, 1,250,000 websites, and 5,080,000 recipes (although, I'm not sure what would actually be the difference between a "foodie" recipe and a regular recipe), and even the definition yields 549,000 results. There are as many definitions for the word "foodie" as there are types of individuals who proclaim to be one. According to one site, the importance of the word is more marketing than anything else. We need to develop an understanding of these definitions to help us gauge exactly what foodie means. Its meaning is important to the context of this book and the possibility of renewing the food system for a number of reasons—the main one being the potential buying power of the foodie. Can that power be great enough to change our food system? Another reason is the association of the word. Does the self-proclamation of a foodie alienate them from the masses? Can we eventually make the masses foodies?

The percentage of foodies seems to be growing every day, but the fact is, according to Marion Nestle, they still only amount to about 20% of the population. Yet, according to Pollan and Hirschberg, the organic sector of the food market is only 3–5%. Based on one "foodie" definition, these numbers should be equal. That being said, Nestle's percentage is based on one particular definition of "foodie" and so these numbers might not need to mesh depending on that particular definition.

The big noise surrounding "foodies," as of late, has been the push back from self-proclaimed foodies regarding the elitist moniker these descriptions bring to the table. Foodies claim: "we are not elitists, and as the local food movement moves forward and our numbers grow they will prove it to everyone." This is a paraphrase from a speech I heard at a recent conference. We'll see whether that will ring true and whether foodies can shed their elitist association. What we do know is that, for the last fifteen years, the local food movement has achieved momentous traction built on the marketing of "Vote with Your Fork" and "Know Your Farmer" campaigns. This approach from the ground up has been, and still is, quite successful. The movement has definitely entered into the mainstream, and most people are at least aware of the cause, even if they are not a part of it.

THE "FOODIE" FACTOR

Before we get into the varying definitions of "foodie" we should understand that, regardless of its exact definition, it is a descriptor of a group of people who have similar traits, such as yuppie, hippie, and preppie before it. Each of these groups has their own stigma or stereotype associated with them. Hippies have a carefree attitude, love everybody, and wear flowers in their hair, or if you don't like them, hippies smell bad, smoke a lot of pot, and don't pay their taxes. A preppie wears bright pink and green, multiple-collared shirts, goes sailing, and goes by Muffy and Biff. A yuppie is a young person who drives a fancy car, wears all the best clothes, and flashes his or her money around to make sure everybody sees it. At least these are the stereotypes shown in the movies, and we all know the movies "accurately" represent any particular stereotype, right? In actuality, a lot of these groups have now blended together, there are yippies or huppies, and, well, you get the picture.

What It Was

Ironically, the inception of the term "foodie" in the early eighties was as an alternative to the original descriptor "gourmet" because of that word's connotation of superiority.[122] It started as a term referring to a wider population of food lovers and since has developed a connection with elitism. Whether it is deserved or not completely depends on which application you choose to follow. The fact that it was coined to incorporate the newly found love of food from the masses over the gourmands, or the original food elitist, makes it that much more ironic. Whatever the initial concept was meant to be, the term has definitely obtained an overtone of exclusivity with the majority of the population. One bit of proof is that foodies are now writing articles commenting on the lack of elitism in the foodie world.

Basically, elitists are perceived as a group of people who feel they are better than everyone else, and because they have more knowledge, they should be treated more favorably. Now this may or may not be true, but the reality is that in America we tend to revolt against the elitist, or at least the openly elitist. Our culture just doesn't like to be told what to do. If there is a group that claims this is the best squash in the city or you can only eat heirloom tomatoes from this one farmer for two weeks in July, it generally turns off most people. Sometimes it's the way in which the information is passed on that can elicit the negative reaction. We've talked about this before. If we force the "only one way" approach on people, then they will automatically resist. The elitist tag is bad for the foodies because they are a large part of the food movement, and it will be more difficult to get others involved if it is deemed selective, snobbish, or stuffy.

With that, let's look at this elitist connotation that the word "foodie" brings to the table. The term "foodie" is applied to a group of like-minded people who share a passion for food. Regardless of the exact definition, knowing that opens you up to the image this group has in public opinion, which currently is one of elitism.

Merriam-Webster defines *elitism* as: 1) leadership, or rule by an *elite*; 2) the selectivity of the elite; *especially*: snobbery—*elitism* in choosing new members; 3) consciousness of being or belonging to an elite.[123]

The *Free Online Dictionary* defines *elitism* as: 1) The belief that certain persons or members of certain classes or groups deserve favored treatment by virtue of their perceived superiority, as in intellect, social status, or financial resources; 2) a. The sense of entitlement enjoyed by such a group or class; b. Control, rule, or domination by such a group or class.[124]

And lastly, *The New Urban Dictionary* has some wonderful potential definitions, but I will just list the latest one for *elitism* because it was humorously enlightening: "A term used by stupid people to describe smart people who speak in complete sentences."[125]

Let's look at a few definitions of "foodie," including the social view from *The Urban Dictionary*. (For a term such as this, the social interpretation might be the most important.)
1) *Merriam-Webster Online*: a person having an avid interest in the latest *food* fads.[126]

2) *The Free Online Dictionary* states: 1) a person having an enthusiastic interest in the preparation and consumption of good food; 2) a person devoted to refined sensuous enjoyment (especially good food and drink).[127]

Some other Google searches include:

1) refined sensuous enjoyment.[128]

2) "foodie" is an informal term for a particular class of aficionado of food and drink. The word was coined in 1981 by Paul Levy and Ann Barr, who used it in the title of their 1984 book *The Official Foodie Handbook.*[129]

3) a person with a special interest or knowledge of food, a gourmet.[130]

4) A person who spends a keen amount of attention and energy on knowing the ingredients of food and the proper preparation of food, and finds great enjoyment in top-notch ingredients and exemplary preparation. A foodie is not necessarily a food snob, only enjoying delicacies and/or food items difficult to obtain and/or expensive foods; though, that is a variety of "foodie."[131]

UNDERSTANDING FOODIES

In his article "The Rise—and—Fall of a Foodie," Dave Mulder did an excellent job covering this very topic, including the urban dictionary definitions and how they had changed over the years. A number of leading food activists have been speaking out lately regarding the term and its snobbish associations. Eric Schlosser comments on how the true elitism in the food world resides not in the foodies but in the controllers of Big Ag. "It gets the elitism charge precisely backward. America's current system of food production—overly centralized and industrialized, overly controlled by a handful of companies . . . . It is one more sign of how the few now rule the many."[132] Schlosser basically calls out the individuals clamoring that foodies are elitist and not representative of a food system that the people truly desire. Nicolette Hahn Niman of Niman Ranch, a vegetarian married to one of the premier ranchers in our country growing meat the right way, comments in direct response to an attacking elitist "foodie" article by B.R. Myers that the food movement is in direct response to the industrial system: "America's food movement emphasizes not only mindful consumption but also reducing waste, conserving natural resources, and respecting the people and animals involved in food production." [133]You could say that, as Americans in the food movement, we are pushing back against the exclusivity of the industrial food system. Both articles make eloquent points to remove the elitist adjective from the "foodie" name, but neither really defines what a foodie is.

Foodie.com is one of the million-plus sites that come up in a Web search and defines a "foodie" as:

> On the *curriculum vitae* of a Foodie, "eating" is listed as a hobby. The Foodie lives to eat, and to eat to live is definitive boredom. A true Foodie clings to all things culinary. From soup to nuts, a Foodie seeks out the fun stuff about fine fare, along with the arcane, the academic, the in-depth, and the latest. To find the perfect cheese or the best macaroon recipe is life's work.[134]

There are a lot more examples of the ultimate "foodie" definition out there, and I will not go into them all. I would like to make an important distinction however. A chef is not a foodie. A server, maitre'd, bartender—none of these are foodies. A restaurant critic is not a foodie, neither is a farmer—though I think that could be debatable. You might be screaming at the book right now, and I can understand that, but I think it is very important to distinguish between these roles.

What It Means

To me a foodie is a combination of all these descriptions. Here is what I've put together as my definition:

> *A foodie is a person who has such a passion for food that their hobby is to know everything there is to know about food. They follow restaurant trends, openings, and closings, chef moves. Chances are they have a blog and spend unpaid hours writing about food. In fact, they are probably in a web of like-minded bloggers through which they share information. Bottom line: They are people who love food. They eat to enjoy, not just to subsist, and they are made up of all kinds, from kids to seniors, across all demographics and races.*

We have reached a new age in this condensed world, and information is in the air around us. If we want to know about the coolest root-beer-flavored green, olasante, like I tasted this weekend for the first time, a quick Internet search and it's at your fingertips. The next step might entail finding a cool store that has it, a chef that makes it, or just finding a recipe for it. Regardless, "foodie" describes those individuals who have a passion about food. They are different from those in the food world who turn this same passion into a career, because those in the food world are supposed to have that passion. They do this for a living. Are there those in the industry who do not have this passion? Yes. And are there foodies who are overtly obnoxious about what they're eating and where they've been? Yes. They are a large reason for the elitist moniker to begin with.

The recent local food movement, the one which a good portion of these foodies have helped to nurture, and its related perceived cost increases have unfortunately earned the elitist tag given by the masses of people who might not fully understand the motivations. Until we can make the right food affordable to everyone, we will not be able to turn everybody into a foodie. Maybe that's not realistic; but, even a very large portion of the population adopting the attitudes, missions, and passions of foodies would be outstanding. By my definition above, the more foodies we can get, the better chance we have of feeding our children real food and giving them the opportunity to become a foodie themselves. The industrial system relies on a lack of interest from the public for knowing where their food comes from. This resistance to foodie-ism that our culture has developed is really an overt act of shooting ourselves in the foot. In general, we don't want to know how that pork lived or died, and the disdain for that kind of information/insight is killing us.

That is one reason why the role of the chef has the power to elicit real change quickly. Does it really matter whether a foodie is considered elitist or not? In the interest of furthering the local food movement, yes, that matters; but in terms of making a serious dent in the companies controlling the food system, no, it doesn't. Yet, if we define a "foodie" as one who craves knowledge for what they are eating, I say we can never have enough foodies. We can't stop cultivating that interest until everybody has developed that respect, that reverence for what they are eating.

Final tāyst

Conclusion
Chefs Can Save the World

My purpose for writing this book was not just to tell the story of greening my restaurant; but, hopefully to show other restaurateurs that it can be done, that it needs to be done, even on a shoestring budget. Green needs to happen. More importantly, I wanted to prove that even if you're not into tree-hugging, saving the environment, or protecting the earth, it is good business. I attempted to demonstrate the connections in our community between the food system and some of the societal issues we face. I wanted to show how these connections drive the way in which we live and, as a result, the state of the world around us. I think it's obvious that the health of the environment, which includes the health of humans, is evident not just in the quantity, but the quality of the food produced. By sharing the stories of my journey, my goal was to touch on these issues without inundating you with data or repetition. I felt that my experiences, married with the information, would be more beneficial to you. My intention was to give you practical ways to apply the information, and hopefully to motivate you to do something about the direction in which our restaurant operations and our food system (and, in turn our country, and the world) are heading. The same issues you see in the paper every day—health care, national security, the economy, the environment, hunger, and disappearing renewable resources—are what we've been addressing. This isn't just about tree-hugging, fancy-food tasting, or government bashing as ways to distract you from your already hectic business. This stuff matters globally but comes to roost at each and every back door as well.

In order to survive, we must be able to produce food—the right food. We have to return to the days in which we were able to be self-sufficient. That doesn't mean we have to be completely and solely self-supporting, importing nothing, only that we could function that way if needed. For as long as we rely on other countries to produce our food, the less chance we have to be a safe and secure nation. The key to a sustainable future lies within our ability to continue producing nutritious food from the healthy earth that is around us, the earth in our communities. Leading food activist Dr. Vandana Silva states: "The future of our world depends on how we steward our land, soil, water, and seeds and pass them on to future generations."[135] While that statement applies to the world at large, I think it resonates more on the community level. By building sustainable communities, we can start to strengthen the pillars that make up a sustainable world.

In my eyes the connections we have been discussing are too obvious to deny or debate. I almost get upset that I didn't uncover this information earlier. After all, I am a passionate chef who loves food. In fact, I am surprised that even the basics about the importance of knowing where your food comes from were not covered in culinary school. The statement "know where your food comes from" holds different implications now than it did when I was in school. It shows how far the local food movement has come. School did stress the importance of knowing your food, the details, the history, and how to prepare it, but discussions about building relationships with your farmers were not part of the lesson. Today that means building a relationship with those who produce, cultivate, harvest, raise, or capture your food. This, fortunately, has changed. Culinary schools and universities are now integrating the importance of sustainable farming into their programs. Remember, this is a new deal. In a world driven by fads and trends, the local movement trend is on the downside. You're starting to see it in the newspapers, where critics are tired of the "farm-to-everything" titles and it is no longer a selling point for restaurants. It is expected. Hopefully, that means it has moved beyond a trend and that it is becoming a fundamental. Regardless, it still has a long way to go, or, as the voice of the trend dies, so will the movement. Chefs have the ability to keep it alive, to ensure that it's at the foundation of our business, and they should because it's the right way to cook and it's what people want to eat.

Look at the amount of noise still being made by the organic food industry, although, like "Eat Local," it seems to have quieted some from a media perspective. Reports indicate that the industry is growing at a rate of 10% a year, yet it still comprises a mere 4% of the food dollars spent in our country.[136] Even though the sales seem minimal, especially compared to regular food sales, large food production companies and some major grocers are introducing organic lines into their offerings. General Mills, Cargill, and Kraft are all producing organic products. Even Walmart is putting organic product on their shelves. Understand, though many have been beating this drum for years, it is just now reaching the public with force. As you know, even I wasn't always concerned with this.

How did we get so far away from knowing our food? How can we just now be serious about finding out where our food comes from? Is it that it was being hidden from us? Was it that we blindly bought into the dream of a pristine little house on the prairie farm land that we learned about in elementary school? Maybe we didn't realize there was another side to the story. For most people, even now, we don't care to ask. Sadly, we've now reached the point where a lot of people are afraid to ask. I know there was a time when I didn't really think twice about what happened on the farms or where my food was grown—and I dealt with food for a living. I went to school to learn about food. I made my whole life about food. Anyone who has chosen this career has made that same choice.

Though I am being so focused on the right way to farm and may, in fact, have demonized the use of industrial agriculture for the majority of this book, I still know there is a large section of people in the country still in favor of its use. They support genetic modification, artificial agents, and technological know-how because of the allure of maximizing food production for the growing world community. They are banking on the claim that without chemical farming we would not be able to feed the booming populations of the world. For years, chemical or industrial farming has been capable of producing mass quantities of bushels per acre; however, according to a recent lecture by Julian Cribb, the yield percentages have ceased to increase and may actually be in decline. The meat industries have engineered their animals not only to grow meat quickly, but to produce the meat the masses desire at a very affordable rate. Of course they leave out the fact that it takes 16 pounds of grain, 2,400 gallons of water, and a lot of fossil fuel to provide one pound of beef.[137] They argue that organic or natural farming doesn't have the ability to produce enough affordable food to support the populace, yet there are plenty of studies that prove otherwise, including a recent report by the U.N. stating that concentrating on an agroecology as states reinvest in agriculture is the best way to curb increasing food prices.[138]

At some point we have to step back and look at the larger picture. We have to take a holistic view of our food system, and that requires taking a look at society as a whole rather than in parts. The last point on which industrial agriculture stands is that the costs of this type of farming prohibitively exceeds the costs of industrial farming, making it inaccessible to the majority of the population. While that fact, in a restrictive view, is true, the true costs of industrial farming extend beyond just the dollar amount in the grocery store. There are many other far-reaching factors to consider. In order to be truly sustainable we have to have a growing medium that is healthy . . . forever. We have to be able to continue to plant on existing land. Another U.N. report states: "There is now abundant scientific evidence that humanity is living unsustainably. Returning human use of natural resources to within sustainable limits will require a major collective effort." Since the 1980s, human sustainability has implied the integration of economic, social, and environmental spheres to "meet the needs of the present without compromising the ability of future generations to meet their own needs."[139]

Isn't a rule of basic physics that with every action there is an equal and opposite reaction? I firmly believe that we started on this path of chemical farming with the good-hearted intention of ending hunger throughout the world. According to Dr. Robert Beachy, whom I recently heard lecture, this effort was, and still is, the reason for genetic modification. It started with a noble purpose, but I believe the proverbial writing is on the wall. We have obviously gone down a path that is having serious effects on the world around us and in us. I am no skinny rat. I lived on fast food for years, and my body shows it; but look around the next time you are in a grocery store or the coffee shop and take note of the prevailing body

255

types you see. Two-thirds of our country is obese and the related illnesses are contributing to the bankrupting of our health care system. For the first time in years, I feel as though I am actually making headway on my weight. Not because I am exercising or "dieting" (I could never "diet," by the way), but because I have changed my diet—what I eat and how I eat it. In fact, I feel I eat more now than I have in years and my weight is going the other direction. I stopped going to fast-food places and I stopped eating processed junk—for the most part. We don't have to be perfect. There is nothing wrong with junk food in moderation. It is okay to swing through the drive-thru every once in a while. The problem lies in the fact that our society is just too busy nowadays with two-job households or single-parent households, and we fall back on this option too often. To say the answer is to cut this out permanently is unrealistic. It is quite likely I will visit a fast-food place again in the future. It is not about being obedient all the time. It is about making the right choices when you have the opportunity. Or, for me, putting my money where my mouth is and starting an organic fast food chain. Bringing both worlds together.

Ideally, if the chefs who control the development of all this snack food we Americans are in love with start to use real food, less processed, more nutritious junk food is possible. I know it sounds like an oxymoron, but it's really only "junk" because it isn't made with real ingredients. All the same, fast-food restaurants that are healthy, affordable, and serve local organic product are possible. There is nothing intrinsically wrong with a burger and fries on occasion. What's wrong is all the unnatural stuff we put in them to make them fast and cheap. If America doesn't want to change, we, the chefs, should change it for them.

I have kids, and even though we are teaching them about where food comes from, they still see McDonald's and scream for Chicken McNuggets. Honestly, a lot of it is driven by that damned Ronald and his goofy commercials and toy giveaways. The weird part about it is my kids have eaten there maybe four or five times in their lives. We teach them that the food that is used at these restaurants is processed—bad for you and the environment—and that it will make you unhealthy. Just recently we were going to a *local* burger joint (doing fast food the right way) and my oldest daughter was telling me about her first Krystal experience while at a friend's house. We were talking about where the meat came from, and the Krystal experience came up. She knew she wasn't supposed to eat the fast-food burger, but didn't want to be impolite at the house where she was playing. She also knew that it would be rude to say her daddy doesn't let her eat that because it's not real food. *Hahaha.* She is pretty smart. She handled it the right way. Every once in a while is okay. Most people don't understand the difference between the local burger joint we visited and the fast-food place. What does that say? It is hard to believe that the majority of people in our country really don't grasp that fast food is bad for them, but that really is the case. People just don't know where their food comes from or bother to inspect the nutritional information. One of the major obstacles we face in our fight to change the food system is that the key to change is getting people to have a vested interest in their food. But the majority of people who truly need this information will not get it, and most of the rest don't want to know. To me, the hardest battle of all is getting the information to the people who need it most.

It's difficult not to regurgitate the words of Pollan, Nestle, Schlosser, Kenner, etc., because they have done an excellent job of not only finding the information, but disseminating it to the public. As my wife always reminds me, "Just because you know, it doesn't mean everybody else does." That being said, if you were unaware of what is going on with our food system before reading this, I urge you to go read more to learn and find out what is going on in the world. We can't expect the leaders of our country to change the system for us. Our choices will determine what is grown. We need to rise up and tell the companies growing our food that it is our choice what we eat. We need to stop accepting what is being provided to us and get these companies to supply what we want. Hopefully, the "we" is not just 20% of the population, as Marion Nestle estimates. Hopefully, the "we" reaches beyond the foodies to the masses, and the wake-up call becomes an earthquake of awareness.

However, let's talk reality. This is a great idea. The belief that if we can teach people where their food comes from, it will get them to change their eating habits makes sense! With the release of "Food, Inc." and similar documentaries, as well as books from the aforementioned authors, more people are learning about the state of our food system. But as is evident in the small percentage of sales from the organic food market, not enough people are being reached. We have groups focusing on climate change, pollution, and a number of other environmental factors. We have groups focusing on health and security and animal rights. We have groups focusing on the food system. All these groups need to come together to fight a singular battle. All these issues are connected. There is power in numbers.

I still find it interesting how my focus on local sources for the benefit of my food quality made me realize the benefits that could extend to my community and eventually the world.

Dining green isn't just about saving the planet, it is about saving your community. The planet will be a natural beneficiary, but the real, visible impact will be realized in your own neighborhoods. In order to promote sustainability in a fashion that will be willingly accepted, or even better, desired, we need to prove it can work. It only takes one community to change, to really look at integrating a food system that feeds all the people within that community. I bet then we would see positive effects across the board within one generation. All the ecosystems in the food world have shown the ability to regenerate or replenish their nutrients when given the opportunity. I think a community, being an ecosystem itself, would react in the same way. I bet health problems would decrease, economic situations would improve, and the general morale of the community would be elevated. We could then take that community and use it as a model for other communities throughout the country.

It has taken us two generations to seriously disrupt our ecosystems. Our generation is at a turning point. We can either choose to push our system back in the right direction, or we can sit idly by and watch it be destroyed. And as the Prince of Wales said recently, "How do we respond when faced with the question from our grandchildren: *Why didn't we do something?*"[140] We can start farming, fishing, and living sustainably, or we can leave a planet that will exponentially deteriorate for our children. The next generation is the key to putting our world back on a sustainable path, and dining green is the answer.

Educating people is a great start and definitely part of the solution, but as we've said, people do not care where their food comes from. I cannot count how many times I have had conversations at the bar with well-educated people who love

259

what we are doing but shudder to think we served a cow that had a name. I am sorry but when the twelve-year-old daughter of one of your farmers names one of her new herd after you, the relationship represented by that honor has to be a good thing. My response to them is always the same: How can that gross you out? How can you believe in what we are doing (which you prove that you do by spending money at the restaurant), and not want to know about the beef? That cow—Jerebob—was treated with love for its entire life, and its afterlife, for that matter. Is that not the ultimate form of respect and care for an animal whose sole purpose is to mow the grass and then feed people? It is exactly the same as knowing where your vegetables come from—something everyone wants to know—yet no one is grossed out about a carrot with a name.

Educating the children is a better choice. In fact, we have a better chance of being effective with education by focusing on teaching our children and letting them spread the word. Youth truly have the ability to enact significant change. We can teach them the difference between good and bad, the truth about where food comes from, and how it is grown or raised. This knowledge would naturally start to reverse the increasing trends of obesity and diabetes in our kids. In successful school gardens across the country, the children not only attack the veggies they have helped grow with delight and excitement, they go home and ask their parents for these veggies to be served at the dinner table. The hope is that the reaction we will get from those parents is for their diets to change as well. As their diets change so does their demand, and, eventually, what is supplied in stores. Unfortunately, as I explained before, the majority of the people we need to teach are not going to get this information if we don't make a concerted effort and dramatic changes in our approach.

Let's say we are successful with this plan of youth education. That's a big portion of the battle done. But now we find on the home front the cost of buying this food is more than most of the families can afford, if it is even accessible. We need not only to teach people but provide them with options that are plausible. Healthy food must be financially manageable and obtainable in order to compete on a large scale with industrial food. That being said, it will never be the same price, at least not today or even tomorrow. The question is, how long until healthy food is easily obtainable? And, can it happen before it's too late? This is where a redirection of subsidies would make sense. Actually, that alone would cause a quicker leveling of the cost of the different food systems since subsidies are one of the main factors in the cheapness of industrial food.

There is one way that always affects change without "what-ifs" and potentialities. There is one driving force that doesn't rely on legislation, policy, and hope. That is the bottom line. Corporations making millions or billions of dollars typically operate at low profit margins. They make their money on pennies, and by changing the direction of some of the pennies we can force the companies to change their operations. The food industry is estimated to sell almost $1.2 trillion worth of goods in 2011. Of those trillion-plus dollars, 50% is spent on food eaten outside of the home.[141] That means restaurants, cars, vending machines, and coffee shops—you can probably throw in mini-marts and gas stations as well—are raking in our disposable income. Who controls most of this money? Chefs, kitchen managers, and food buyers.

Chefs are the key to a sustainable future. Many people put their faith in us to make the meals they purchase to be nutritious. That trust is probably what fans the belief that fast food or processed food is okay to eat often. Most people think that there is no way a business would knowingly serve food that is detrimental to their health. As chefs, it is our passion to put the best food on the table. It just so happens that the best food is probably grown, raised, or caught in a sustainable manner. We have developed good momentum in the farm-to-table movement within the upscale/fine-dining and independent casual sector of the restaurant industry. Unfortunately, only a small part of the population consistently eats in these establishments. They are also the ones most likely to be aware of the importance of knowing your food. We, as chefs, need to band together in our purchasing decisions and start buying safe, healthy food. The way we can successfully do that is by integrating education that is focused on the upcoming chefs and cooks. This will be even more powerful if we combine it with education at the primary level.

If you are unfamiliar with how the restaurant world works, it is a web of networking. Young chefs either work their way up or go to school—the benefit of school being they obtain a wealth of knowledge at a quicker pace. They move from restaurant to restaurant, learning from different chefs as they go. Some of the cooks coming up now might be fortunate enough to be working for chefs who are buying in a sustainable manner. They are getting the opportunity to see how it is done, taste the differences in the product, and hopefully learn that these purchases make a larger difference beyond the kitchen door. Moreover, they are getting the experience of how to build a local food infrastructure and make that work for a restaurant. For those who are in school, I can only hope the books addressing the food system are required reading. The newly introduced sustainable restaurant courses are a great step in the right direction. The courses should also integrate lessons on how to ask the right questions, how to source local product, and the environmental impacts of the different styles of farming.

Right now, local, sustainable food is primarily in upscale establishments as I said, but many more cooks move through these places while training than actually end up running them. These types of establishments are a small percentage of the restaurant industry. Most of these cooks will not end up in the same restaurants in which they learned; but, those restaurants are responsible for turning loose into the industry those who will become corporate chefs, personal chefs, caterers, hospital and other institutional kitchen staff, culinary instructors, etc. If the learning they received in the field mimicked what was being taught in the culinary schools, we could realistically have a functional and complete farm-to-fork system by the end of the next generation. If these cooks are learning how to buy and utilize their entire product, they are also learning how to make food profitable. They are battling the one valid argument against sustainable food right now: cost. They are learning the skills to be able to make sustainable food work.

Now that we have a workforce dedicated to purchasing sustainable product, we need an infrastructure that can support it. As it stands, in most locations the demand is greater than the supply. One big positive movement I am seeing just in the last year or two is an influx of younger farmers going back to the land. These are young entrepreneurs who see the potential to make money on the farm again. But they also see that the profit potential is in sustainable farming. As with most businesses, farming has evolved to require a skill set, not just in farming, but in self-promotion as well. In order to be successful, they are forced to establish themselves in their communities. It has become a part of the business.

The other hindrance is the cost of getting started. Very often I am talking to young couples or individuals who are trying to acquire land in order to start farming. It is hard for them to compete with real estate developers seeing the next big suburb. For the existing land owners, most of them probably ex-farmers, it is hard to fault them for selling to the highest bidder. They need to make as much money as they can. The story behind all this is that most of the ex-farmers who are selling and getting out of industrial farming are doing so because it isn't profitable. The industrial farmers are looking for a way out and the organic farmers are looking for a way in. Is that not the best proof we have seen so far? If the arguments from these industrial proponents were valid, would we not see the opposite occurring? The industrial proponents' answer to this is that we need less people to farm with continued advancement in industrial technique. Former secretary of agriculture Earl Butz's "Get Big or Get Out" program has pushed our agriculture to the point that farmers comprise less than 1% of the population, with only 200,000 folks producing 85% of the food in the country. The last couple of years have also produced record profits for these farms according to current Secretary of Agriculture Tom Vilsack.[142] Since 2004, three of those years have been the most profitable of the last thirty-five years.[143] Although forecasts for this year are now down due to the poor spring weather.

It is true that advancements are making it easier to farm with less labor, making these farms profitable. I just don't believe people are so willing to give up farms (most of which have been in families for generations) so easily, and it is obvious that only a very small number of individuals were able to "get big." It seems to me that farmers would need a pretty big reason to give up their land, such as lack of profitability. Oh, and in all these years of record profit for big agriculture, the industrial farms still received a majority of the subsidies. The other downside from less labor on the farm is that we took more jobs out of a market that is at the highest unemployment rate in years. Somehow we as a society have deemed the most important job in our country—feeding people—unprofessional. We've spent years convincing them to get off of their farms and get professional jobs in the city, yet we don't have enough jobs for them. We have lost the experiential knowledge of how to farm –knowledge passed down through generations of family farmers. I wonder if we can ever get back the knowledge of the subtle nuances of insight from previous generations about the best way to farm their land. Hopefully, this trend reverses. Hopefully, we can start to rebuild what is probably the most important industry we have, with young farmers using sustainable methods. That will increase the supply of nutritious healthy food, but it will not be the sole solution.

This brings us back to chefs being the answer to a sustainable future. Increasing the number of farmers will help increase supply and get us going in the right direction. Educating the masses will help drive demand, but that will only take us so far. To truly be successful in the fight against industry, we must get industry to realize they need to change. If we can get just 30% of the next generation of chefs outside of independent, fine dining places to buy in a sustainable manner, I think we have a legitimate way to force the hand of the industrial machines. Think about the pennies these machines run on. A 30% change in food purchases would cause these major companies to change the way they do business. Their profits would be hurt enough to influence their decisions about farming sustainably or using product from sustainable farms. It would at least raise red flags at the board meetings.

I will say it again: $1.2 trillion, 50% of which is controlled by chefs! These are the numbers that hold the power. People don't want to be told what to eat, but they don't want to have to think about their food either. We can imagine all the beautiful fantasies of awareness we want, but here is the reality: being truly informed requires more effort than most have the time or energy to give. The food companies know this, and they capitalize on it. At the "Future of Food" conference presented by *The Washington Post* this year, Susan Crockett from General Mills blatantly confirmed that argument. General Mills is already starting to move toward healthier products without promoting that fact. Their method is to slowly decrease the salt or sugar in an item milligram by milligram. Each year they decrease the sugar in a product by one milligram so the palates of the masses can't detect a change in their favorite cereal, Hot Pocket, or whatever. Eventually, they will be making a product for the future that is significantly healthier. This shows these companies are listening to the public. It also shows they are willing to change. That alone makes the power of chefs controlling the $600 billion that much more effective.

The profit margins of these companies vary from 1%, as with Maple Leaf Foods, all the way to the 14% of PepsiCo. The majority, however, see 6–10% with the average being around 8%. Unilever is 10%, Heinz is around 9%, Kraft is 6%, General Mills is between 8% and 9.5% (depending on the reporting source), Groupe Danone is 9.9%, and ConAgra is 8.9%. (These numbers were compiled from an average of the statistics found from a variety of sources.)[144] Some of these companies are 100% food sales, but a good portion diversify in some direction or another. The average food sales for these companies is about 75%. Using those numbers, around 6% of the profits for the leading food production companies are directly related to food sales. The formulas for the exact profit breakdown are probably much more complex than my cook's math. The wow factor is that a nominal change in food sales will affect the bottom line. If we, as chefs, can come together to demand the right product, the ripple effects will change the food system as we know it. If one company can't provide what we demand, another one will. Competition will benefit our cause. Look at the expansion of earth-friendly disposables that have found their way into the distribution companies in the last couple of years.

We are still years away from getting back to the days of the expert butcher on the corner, and bringing family meals around the dinner table again. Food production companies are integral to providing the lifestyle our society is accustomed to having. We must like this way of life because we are continuing to move it forward. We need to fix the food system in a manner in which it meshes with the way the masses want to live and is still sustainable. We want food fast and easy and cheap. That can be done, and be done sustainably. Chefs developing the recipes and ideas that fit into this system now need to be integrating organic products, sourcing locally where possible, and utilizing sustainable practices. We need to ensure that the next round of chefs making their way into the restaurant industry believe in making those choices work within the system. Food buyers out there need to request these options from the production companies.

The small percentage we start with will turn into a larger percentage as the next generation enters the workforce. The change will happen progressively, but exponentially. As more products are requested by more people, more will be produced, and, in turn, more variety will become available. The people will purchase what we give them. We can give them real food, good food, the right food.

Every culinary school must teach sustainable dining. Every young chef coming up through the ranks should know the origins of their food and all the residual environmental effects of the production of their food. We have already seen the change starting in my generation, and we can only hope that it continues with the voraciousness with which it started. If you combine all the cooks of my generation who have made change with the ones hopefully learning sustainability from the next generation, I think 30% is a very conservative number of those who will be advocating for the effort. As our numbers grow, so will our power. Chefs have the power to make food companies listen. We have the power to make food companies change how they are operating. When we stand up and start putting our money where our mouths are, sustainable methods and products will be implemented. When one or two companies show sustainable food-related profit, the rest will follow.

The most important trickle-down from raising our collective voices will be the increased awareness of our diners. If restaurants truly drive the food trends, which I believe they do, then diners eating sustainable food will leave the restaurants in search of sustainable food. The cookbooks and talk shows will begin showing primarily green food methods.

The Food Network will host green dining shows . . . . Who knows? Maybe one will be mine! HaHa! People will truly begin to understand how to go about being green in their food choices. That's when we stumble into the benefits on health care and school systems and so on. Maybe we will finally find that we are no longer feeding fast food to hospital patients. (Inconceivable, isn't it?)

There are so many possibilities and solutions for making this movement work. I don't know why it is so difficult to see that the wheels have come off the bus and we are careening out of control in the wrong direction. Maybe one of the biggest benefits to dining green is the evolution toward living in a sustainable manner—a greater push toward viewing sustainability from all points of view: food, water, waste, and energy. We can't force people to follow this path, but we will be much more persuasive if we give them room to find their own place in the system, to decide what level of commitment works for them. We can raise the next generation of business owners to be sustainable. Obviously, I am invested in the food system and believe it is the place to start because it touches the largest number of components of this issue. Changing the food system will put a great dent in all the other environmental concerns. With a little push the next generation will start to do it on their own. With the right type of encouragement and guidance, they will take the reins and really expand this revolution. When I started on this path, writing about how to do this was the last thing I ever expected. The more time and energy I invested in this work, the more I realized that, though I have started walking, I needed to be talking. This doesn't have to be an overwhelming process. This doesn't have to be an impossible process. If you take baby steps and start small, you will end up doing more than you think you can do. All you need to start with is a little effort and a bit more passion for making a difference.

Are my ideas *the* answer? I don't know. I feel they are. I have read most of the books and seen most of the documentaries. However, I am no expert, or at least I don't feel that way. I know people seem to be really interested in what we do at *tāyst*. I do not feel we have blazed trails necessarily, but we have definitely opened some doors in our region. I want to lead others to and through those doors. I know there is so much more to learn, not just about cooking, but also about the environmental issues we face as a community, as a society, and as a people. Every time we do something new, we learn more, and maybe we can make it easier for the next restaurant. I want to share my stories because I want to make green accessible, especially the food. If you don't want to get certified green, or even go green at all, at least cook sustainably—because even if you don't have kids, someone you know does. When you strip away all of the politics, the power, and the money. it really is all about the children and leaving this planet a better place for them.

Appendix A

Tables

Table 1. Food and Agricultural Organization's most recent food prices.

January 2011

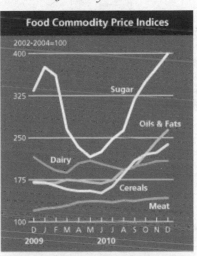

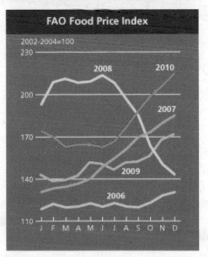

FAO Food Price Index Data

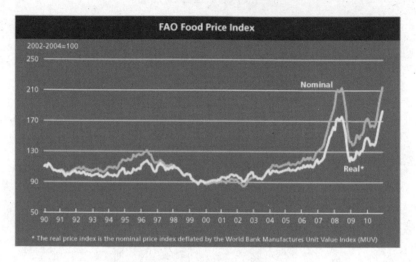

FAO Food Price Index

2002-2004=100

Nominal

Real*

90 91 92 93 94 95 96 97 98 99 00 01 02 03 04 05 06 07 08 09 10

* The real price index is the nominal price index deflated by the World Bank Manufactures Unit Value Index (MUV)

FAO Food Price Index Deflated Data

		Food Price Index [1]	Meat [2]	Dairy [3]	Cereals [4]	Oils and Fats [5]	Sugar [6]
				FAO food price index			
2000		90	94	95	85	68	116
2001		92	94	107	86	68	123
2002		90	90	82	95	87	98
2003		98	99	95	98	101	101
2004		111	111	123	107	112	102
2005		115	113	135	103	104	140
2006		122	107	128	121	112	210
2007		154	112	212	167	169	143
2008		191	128	220	238	225	182
2009		152	118	142	174	150	257
2009	December	172	120	216	171	169	334
2010	January	174	124	202	170	169	376
	February	170	125	191	164	169	361
	March	163	129	187	158	175	265
	April	165	135	204	155	174	233
	May	164	137	209	155	170	216
	June	163	137	203	151	168	225
	July	167	134	198	163	174	247
	August	177	138	193	185	192	263
	September	188	137	198	208	198	318
	October	199	140	203	220	220	349
	November	206	141	208	223	243	373
	December	215	142	208	238	263	398

1 **Food Price Index**: Consists of the average of 6 commodity group price indices mentioned above weighted with the average export shares of each of the groups for 2002-2004: in total 55 commodity quotations considered by FAO commodity specialists as representing the international prices of the food commodities noted are included in the overall index.

2 **Meat Price Index**: Consists of 3 poultry meat product quotations (the average weighted by assumed fixed trade weights), 4 bovine meat product quotations (average weighted by assumed fixed trade weights), 2 pig meat product quotations (average weighted by assumed fixed trade weights), 1 ovine meat product quotation (average weighted by assumed fixed trade weights): the 4 meat group average prices are weighted by world average export trade shares for 2002-2004.

3 **Dairy Price Index**: Consists of butter, SMP, WMP, cheese, casein price quotations; the average is weighted by world average export trade shares for 2002-2004.

4 **Cereals Price Index**: This index is compiled using the grains and rice price indices weighted by their average trade share for 2002-2004. The Grains Price Index consists of International Grains Council (IGC) wheat price index, itself average of 9 different wheat price quotations, and 1 maize export quotation; after expressing the maize price into its index form and converting the base of the IGC index to 2002-2004. The Rice Price Index consists of 3 components containing average prices of 16 rice quotations: the components are Indica, Japonica and Aromatic rice varieties and the weights for combining the three components are assumed (fixed) trade shares of the three varieties.

5 **Oil and Fat Price Index**: Consists of an average of 11 different oils (including animal and fish oils) weighted with average export trade shares of each oil product for 2002-2004.

6 **Sugar Price Index**: Index form of the International Sugar Agreement prices with 2002-2004 as base.

Appendix B
Recommended Reading
and Resources

These are just a few of the many books out there regarding sustainability, agriculture, food policy, and environmental issues, but they are a great start. Many of the authors listed below have multiple books and other selected articles to help mold your understanding of the intricacies of the food system. There are also authors like Wendell Barry, Joan Dye Gussow, and Fred Kirschenman who have been the leaders of the sustainable agriculture movement.

Books

Anthelme Brillat-Savarin, Jean, *The Physiology of Taste*, Counterpoint, 2000

Cribb, Julian, *The Coming Famine: The Global Food Crisis and What We Can Do to Avoid It*, Univ. of California Press, 2010

Greenberg, Paul, *Four Fish: The Future of the Last Wild Food*, Penguin, 2010

Halweil, Brian, *Eat Here: Homegrown Pleasures in a Global Supermarket*, WW Norton, 2004

Hirschberg, Gary, *Stirring It Up: How to Make Money and Save the World*, Hyperion, 2008

Imhoff, Daniel (editor), *The CAFO Reader: The Tragedy of Industrial Animal Factories*, University of California Press, 2010

Kamp, David, *The United States of Arugula: The Sun Dried, Col Pressed, Dark Roasted, Extra Virgin Story of the American Food Revolution*, Broadway Books, 2006

Kingsolver, Barbara, *Animal, Vegetable, Miracle: A Year of Food Life*, Harper Perennial, 2007

Lappe, Anna, *Diet for a Hot Planet: The Climate Crisis at the End of Your Fork and What You Can Do About It*, Bloomsbury USA, 2010

Lovins, L. Hunter and Boyd Cohen, *Climate Capitalism: Capitalism in the Age of Climate Change*, Hill and Wang, 2011

Mas Masumoto, David, *Wisdom of the Last Farmer: Harvesting Legacies from the Land*, Simon and Schuster, 2007

Nestle, Marion, *What to Eat*, North Point Press, 2006

Niman, Nicolette Hahn, *Righteous Porkchop*, William Morrow, 2009

Pollan, Michael, *In Defense of Food: An Eater's Manifesto*, Penguin Press, 2008

Roberts, Paul, *The End of Food*, Mariner Books, 2008

Salatin, Joel, *Holy Cows and Hog Heaven: The Food Buyers Guide to Farm Friendly Food*, Polyface, 2004

Schlosser, Eric, *Chew On This: Everything You Don't Want to Know About Fast Food*, Houghton Mifflin, 2006

Schlosser, Eric, *Fast Food Nation, The Dark Side of the American Meal*, Harper Perennial, 2002

Pollan, Michael, *Food Rules: An Eater's Manual*, Penguin Press, 2011

Pollan, Michael, *The Omnivores Dilemna: A Natural History of Four Meals*, Penguin Press, 2006

Smith, Jeffery M., *Seeds of Deception: Exposing Industry and Government Lies About the Safety of Genetically Engineered Foods You're Eating*, Yes Books, 2003

Wasnick, Brian, *Mindless Eating: Why We Eat More Than We Think*, Bantam Books, 2006

Weber, Karl, Ed., *Food, Inc.: How Industrial Food is Making Us Sicker, Fatter, and Poorer—and What You Can Do About It*, Public Affairs, 2009

Winne, Mark, *Food Rebels, Guerrilla Gardeners, and Smart Cookin' Mamas: Fighting Back in an Age of Industrial Agriculture*, Beacon Press, 2010

Documentaries

Food Inc.

Foodmatters

The Future of Food: You Are What You Eat

King Corn

Grow

Tapped

The Real Dirt on Farmer John

The World According to Monsanto

The GMO Trilogy

Bad Seed: The Truth About Our Food

One Man, One Cow, One planet

Dirt! The Movie

The End of the Line

Chow Down

A River of Waste: The Hazardous Truth About Factory Farms

Ripe for Change

Author Biography

Jeremy Barlow discovered the food business early while spending summers on Nantucket Island. After graduating from Vanderbilt University with a degree in psychology, Jeremy attended the Culinary Institute of America. At CIA he worked with some of the world's best chefs and graduated with honors, receiving the Francis L. Roth award of excellence for academic and extracurricular performance. He interned at the Inn at Blackberry Farm with John Fleer.

After graduation Jeremy returned to Nashville to eventually open his own restaurant. He now operates tayst, serving playful American cuisine, and Sloco, a sandwich shop, both dedicated to sourcing ingredients locally and organically. Jeremy has become an outspoken advocate for responsible practices in restaurant operations. His message is demonstrated in the methods he employs for running his businesses.

Jeremy lives in Nashville with his wife and two daughters.

www.taystrestaurant.com

www.slocolocal.com

NOTES

Introduction

[1] Laurence C. Smith, *The World in 2050*, New York: Dutton 2010, pg 10.

[2] Kelly Brownell and Kenneth E. Warner, "The Perils of Ignoring History: Big Tobacco Played Dirty and Millions Died. How Similar Is Big Food?" *The Milbank Quarterly*, Vol. 87, No. 1, 2009 (pp. 259–294).

[3] Http://www.epa.gov/sustainability/basicinfo.htm.

[4] Http://www.dinegreen.com/.

[5] "GRA Technomic Survey," May 2010, http://restaurantnewsresource.mobi/?p-45979.

Chapter 3

[6] Http://thegovmonitor.com/world news/united_states/farmers-markets-nationwide-increase-more-than-13-percent-in-growth-from-last-year-8026.html.

[7] Http://www.ethylenecontrol.com/about.php.

[8] Http://www.theatlantic.com/food/archive/2011/01/fao-food-price-index-reaches-its-highest-recorded-level/69129.

[9] Thomas Burstyn, *How to Save the World: One Man, One Cow, One Planet*, DVD, Cloud South Films, 2008.

[10] Http://www.sustainabletable.org/issues/ge/.

[11] Michael Pollan, "The Farmer in Chief," *New York Times*, Oct.12, 2008, pg. 8.

[12] " USDA Agricultural Census," http://www.agcensus.usda.gov/Publications/2007/Full_Report/index.asp

[13] "EWG Farm Bill 2007," http://farm.ewg.org/sites/farmbill2007/progdetail1614.php?fips=00000&progcode=farmprog&page=conc.

[14] California Department of Food and Agriculture. "A Food Foresight Analysis of Agricultural Biotechnology: A Report to the Legislature," January 1, 2003. http://www.sustainabletable.org/issues/ge/.
[15] "Emerging Infectious Diseases," http://www.cdc.gov/ncidod/eid/vol5no5/mead.htm.
[16] *How to Save the World.*
[17] Marc Kaufman, "U.S. Genetically Modified Corn Is Assailed," *Washington Post*, Wednesday, November 10, 2004, Page A02, http://www.washingtonpost.com/wp-dyn/articles/A37992-2004Nov9.html.
[18] "USDA Sustainable Agriculture: Definitions and Terms," http://www.nal.usda.gov/afsic/pubs/terms/srb9902.shtml.
[19] Jenna Rae Fearnley, "Effects of Industrial Agriculture of Crops on Water and Soil," http://knol.google.com/k/effects-of-industrial-agriculture-of-crops-on-water-and-soil#.
[20] Elaine R. Ingham, B.A., M.S., Ph.D. "The Soil Foodweb: Its Role in Ecosystem Health," http://www.agroforestry.net/overstory/overstory81.html.
[21] Tom Philpott , "Fork It Over: Food Miles to Go," http://www.grist.org/article/fork-it-over-food-miles-to-go/.
[22] Anup Shah, "Carbon Sinks, Forest and Climate Change," http://www.globalissues.org/article/180/carbon-sinks-forests-and-climate-change.
[23] Tom Philpott, "Can Industrial Agriculture Feed the World," http://www.grist.org/article/can-industrial-agriculture-feed-the-world/.
[24] Brian Halweil, *Eat Here, Reclaiming Homegrown Pleasures in a Global Supermarket*, New York: W.W. Norton & Co., 2004, p. 56–57.
[25] "Living Organic," http://www.living-organic.net/organic-farming.html.
[26] "Consumer Brochure, USDA National Organic Program," http://www.ams.usda.gov/nop/Consumers/brochure.html.
[27] Rebecca M. Litts, "Rejoining Nature and Food Production: An Argument in Support of Sustainable Agriculture," http://www.annualglobalcollegeconference.com/uploads/6/8/9/8/6898942/senior_thesis_-_rebecca_litts.pdf
[28] *How to Save the World.*

[29] Http://www.restaurant.org/research/.

Chapter 4

[30] Mark Bittman, "Rethinking the Meat Guzzler," http://www.nytimes.com/2008/01/27/weekinreview/27bittman.html.
[31] "Food and Water Watch," http://www.foodandwaterwatch.org/food/factoryfarms/.
[32] Http://articles.latimes.com/2011/feb/24/business/la-fi-food-prices-20110224.
[33] The Food and Agriculture Organization of the United Nations "FAO Initiative on Soaring Food Prices," http://www.fao.org/isfp/isfp-home/en/.
[34] Eric Schlosser, *Fast Food Nation*, New York: Harper Perennial, 2005, pg. 3.
[35] "RNCOS Industry Research Solutions 2010 Market Report on Fast Food," http://www.rncos.com/Report/IM014.htm.
[36]
Http://www.fao.org/newsroom/en/news/2006/1000448/index.html.
[37] Http://www.epa.gov/methane/.
[38] Http://www.epa.gov/nitrousoxide/index.html.
[39] Http://www.beefusa.org/thcicattleindustryhistory.aspx.
[40] Richard Robbins, *Global Problems and the Culture of Capitalism*, New York: Prentice Hall, 2010, p.220.
[41] Http://www.sustainabletable.org/issues/environment/.
[42] "Preservation of Antibiotics for Medical Treatment Act," http://webcache.googleusercontent.com/search?q=cache:_mlaLT4M57MJ:www.ucsusa.org/food_and_agriculture/solutions/wise_antibiotics/pamta.html+current+percentage+of+antibiotics+for+animals&cd=9&hl=en&ct=clnk&gl=us&source=www.google.com.
[43] Factory Farm Nation, "How America Turned Its Livestock Farms into Factories," http://documents.foodandwaterwatch.org/FactoryFarmNation-web.pdf
[44] Http://www.nrdc.org/water/pollution/nspills.asp.
[45]
Http://www.fao.org/newsroom/en/news/2006/1000448/index.html.
[46] Http://www.eatwild.com/index.html.

47

Http://www.fsis.usda.gov/Fact_Sheets/Meat_&_Poultry_Labeling_
Terms/index.asp.

Chapter 5

[48] Bruce Barcott, "What's the Catch,"
http://www.onearth.org/article/whats-the-catch?page=2.
[49] "Coastal Zone Pop Method,"
http://sedac.ciesin.columbia.edu/es/papers/Coastal_Zone_Pop_Met
hod.pdf.
[50] Charles Clover, "The End of the Line," DVD,
http://endoftheline.com/film.
[51] Ray Hilborn, "Let Us Eat Fish,"
http://www.nytimes.com/2011/04/15/opinion/15hilborn.html.
[52]

Http://webcache.googleusercontent.com/search?q=cache:RrxkUAH9
7nAJ:www.marine-
conservation.org.uk/marine%2520conservation.html+Unsustainable+
fishing+caused+by+poor+fisheries+management+and+wasteful+destr
uctive+fishing+practices+is+decimating+the+world+fisheries,+marine
+habitats,+and+killing+billions+of+unwanted+fish+and+other+marin
e+animals."&cd=1&hl=en&ct=clnk&gl=us&client=safari.
[53]

Http://wwf.panda.org/about_our_earth/blue_planet/problems/proble
ms_fishing/.
[54]

Http://www.panda.org/about_our_earth/blue_planet/problems/probl
ems_fishing/access_agreements/.
[55] Ibid.
[56]

Http://www.panda.org/about_our_earth/blue_planet/problems/probl
ems_fishing/illegal_fishing/.
[57] Jim Patrick and Rob Benchley, *Scallop Season: A Nantucket
Chronicle*, New York: Autopscot Press, 2002.
[58]Http://www.savingseafood.org/economic-impact/nantucket-bay-
scallop-catch-less-than-half-the-yield-of-yea-3.html.
[59]

Http://www.globalcoral.org/frequently_asked_questions.htm#Wh
at%20are%20the%20consequences%20of%20reef%20morbidity.

[60] Http://chefscollaborative.org/2011/01/25/an-introduction-and-five-farmed-fish/.

[61] Http://www.sciencedaily.com/releases/2011/04/110407092034.htm.

[62] Http://www.thefishsite.com/articles/30/a-technical-opinion-on-the-wild-salmon-farmed-salmon-debate.

[63] Http://www.fishfarmer-magazine.com/news/fullstory.php/aid/1902/Record_increase_in_salmon_prices.html.

[64] Reenita Malhotra, "Sustainable Fish Choices for an Overfished Planet," http://www.greenlivingideas.com.

[65] Http://www.foodandwaterwatch.org/fish/fish-farming/.

[66] Http://www.kona-blue.com /sustainability.php.

[67] Http://chefscollaborative.org/2011/01/25/an-introduction-and-five-farmed-fish/.

[68] Http://tradestandards.org/en/Standard.9.aspx.

[69] Alan Burdick, "Home on the Fish Range," http://www.onearth.org/article/home-on-the-fish-range.

Chapter 6

[70] Michael Pollan, "The Farmer in Chief," *New York Times*, 2008.

[71] Ibid.

[72] Http://www.cspinet.org/nutritionpolicy/nutrition_policy.html#obese.

[73] Http://www.chefann.com.

[74] Http://www.cspinet.org/nutritionpolicy/nutrition_policy.html#obese.

[75] Ibid.

[76] Ibid.

[77] Brian Wasnick, *Mindless Eating: Why We Eat More Than We Think*, New York: Bantam, 2006.

[78] *How to Save the World*.

Chapter 7

[79] Http://www.restaurant.org/research/facts/.

Chapter 8

[80] Http://www.interlockonline.com.
[81] Http://www.dinegreen.com/standards/Energy.html.

Chapter 9

[82] Http://www.dinegreen.com/customers/education.asp,
http://www.dinegreen.com/customers/education.asp.
[83] Http://greenliving.about.com/od/greenathome/a/energy-efficient-air-conditioning.htm.
[84] Http://www.dinegreen.com/standards/Disposables.html.
[85] Ibid.
[86] Ibid.

Chapter 10

[87] Http://www.naturalcandles.com /Articles.asp?id=142.

Chapter 12

[88] Http://www.cflknowhow.org/value-of-cfls.html.
[89] Ibid.
[90] Http://www.energy.gov/energysources/coal.htm.
[91] Http://www.cflfacts.com/.
[92] Http://electronics.howstuffworks.com/led.htm.
[93]

Http://www.carbonfund.org/site/pages/carbon_calculators/category/Assumptions.

Chapter 13

[94] Http://www.dinegreen.com/customers/education.asp.
[95]

Http://www.cbsnews.com/stories/2005/11/09/health/main1029857.s
html#ixzz1Ooq3ZkOB.
[96] Http://www.dinegreen.com/customers/education.asp.
[97] Ibid.

[98] Ibid.

[99] Http://www.smithsonianmag.com/science-nature/plastic.html?c=y&page=1.

[100] Ibid.

[101]

Http://www.goodcleantech.com/2008/08/biotech_firm_grows_plastic_in.php.

[102] Http://www.worldcentric.org/biocompostables/plant-fiber.

Chapter 14

[103] Http://www.dinegreen.com/customers/education.asp.

[104] Http://www.ci.la.ca.us/san/solid_resources/pdfs/FoodWaste.pdf.

[105] Http://www.epa.gov/epawaste/facts-text.htm - chart1.

[106] Http://www.epa.gov/epawaste/basic-solid.htm.

[107] Http://www.stalkmarketproducts.com/myth.html.

[108]

Http://www.epa.gov/waste/conserve/materials/organics/food/index.htm.

[109] Http://www.epa.gov/waste/conserve/materials/organics/food/fd-basic.htm.

[110]

Http://www.sciencedaily.com/releases/2009/11/091124204314.htm.

[111] Http://www.fao.org/news/story/en/item/74192/icode/.

[112]

Http://www.sciencedaily.com/releases/2009/11/091124204314.htm.

[113] Http://www.fao.org/news/story/en/item/74192/icode/.

[114]

Http://www.epa.gov/epawaste/conserve/materials/organics/food/fd-basic.htm.

Chapter 15

[115] Reay Tannahill, *Food in History,* New York: Broadway, 1995.

[116]

Http://www.ams.usda.gov/AMSv1.0/ams.fetchTemplateData.do?template=TemplateS&leftNav=WholesaleandFarmersMarkets&page=WFMFarmersMarketGrowth&description=Farmers%20Market%20Growth&acct=frmrdirmkt.

[117] *How to Save the World.*

Chapter 17

118

http://computingforsustainability.wordpress.com/2009/03/15/vis
ualising-sustainability/.
[119] Http://www.whiteoakpastures.com/index.php?id=21.
120

Http://www.guardian.co.uk/environment/2007/mar/03/travelsenviro
nmentalimpact.transportintheuk.
[121] Http://www.treehugger.com/files/2010/10/global-aviation-
industry-cap-emissions-2020-strengthens-energy-efficiency-
target.php.
[122] Http://www.eatingrealfood.com/articles/the-
rise%E2%80%94and-fall%E2%80%94of-foodie/.

Chapter 18

[123] Http://www.merriam-webster.com /dictionary/elitism.
[124] Http://www.thefreedictionary.com/elitism.
[125] Http://www.urbandictionary.com/define.php?term=elitism.
[126] Http://www.merriam-
webster.com/dictionary/foodie?show=0&t=1315923560.
[127] Http://www.thefreedictionary.com/foodie.
[128] Http://wordnetweb.princeton.edu/perl/webwn.
[129] Http://en.wikipedia.org/wiki/Foodie.
[130] Ibid.
[131] Http://www.urbandictionary.com/define.php?term=foodie.
[132] Http://www.washingtonpost.com/opinions/why-being-a-foodie-
isnt-elitist/2011/04/27/AFeWsnFF_story.html
[133] Http://www.theatlantic.com/life/archive/2011/02/defending-
foodies-a-rancher-takes-a-bite-out-of-b-r-67myers/71416/.
[134] Http://www.foodies.com/misc/foodie.html.

Conclusion

[135] Http://www.vandanashiva.org/?p=605.
[136] Http://www.ota.com/organic/mt/business.html.
[137] Http://www.peta.org/issues/animals-used-for-food/meat-wastes-
natural-resources.aspx.

[138] Http://www.huffingtonpost.com/paula-crossfield/un-ecofarming-feeds-the-world_b_833340.html.

[139] United Nations General Assembly *Report of the World Commission on Environment and Development: Our Common Future.* Transmitted to the General Assembly as an Annex to document A/42/427 - Development and International Co-operation: Environment. Retrieved on: February 15, 2009.

[140] http://washingtonpostlive.com/conferences.

[141] http://www.restaurant.org/research/facts/.

[142] http://washingtonpostlive.com/conferences.

[143] http://www.ers.usda.gov/briefing/farmincome/nationalestimates.htm.

http://seekingalpha.com/article/102103-the-top-10-global-food-producers-an-overview. http://www.foodprocessing.com/top100/.